W9-CER-129

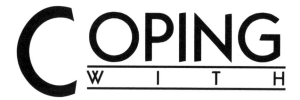

COPING WITH

Drugs and Sports

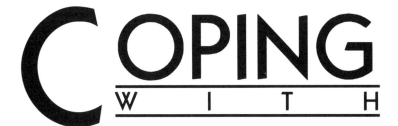

COPING
W I T H

Drugs
and Sports

Elizabeth Ann Nelson

THE ROSEN PUBLISHING GROUP, INC./NEW YORK

Published in 1992 by The Rosen Publishing Group, Inc.
29 East 21st Street, New York, NY 10010

First Edition

Library of Congress Cataloging-in-Publication Data

Nelson, Elizabeth Ann, 1942–
    Coping with drugs and sports / Elizabeth Ann Nelson.
        p.   cm.
    Includes bibliographical references and index.
    Summary: Examines the dangers of drug use in sports, discussing such substances as prescription drugs, alcohol, cocaine, pain relievers, steroids, and tobacco.
    ISBN 0-8239-1342-2
    1. Coping in sports—Juvenile literature.   [1. Coping in sports.
2. Drugs.   3. Drug abuse.]   I. Title.
RC1230.N46   1992
362.29'08'8796—dc20   91-32395
                                                                   CIP
                                                                    AC

Manufactured in the United States of America

To David Nelson-Fischer, my son.

To Cordner and Mary Nelson, my parents.

To Jeannette Rolleri, my mentor.

To Bill and Mary Siegert, my friends.

A B O U T   T H E   A U T H O R ◇

E lizabeth Ann Nelson lives in a cabin full of books in Pacific Grove, California, with her son, David, and their golden retriever, Casey Jones.

Her academic training has included a double major in art and psychology for a BA degree; an MA in Creative Arts Interdisciplinary Studies with Teaching Credentials, and a post-MA dual degree program in psychology and counseling. She has taught at all levels in a variety of schools.

She has written about the arts and personal development through the individuation process. Her book about coping with stress in drugs and sports was approached with the same value: to help others attain their personal best.

Contents

CHAPTER 1

Athletes Fail and Die from Drugs

A teenage athlete was asked, "What do you want to know about drugs and sports?

He might have asked which drugs would be best to improve his performance or to build his strength and endurance, or which drugs could be used for pain, injuries, and inflammation. Instead, lines of worry creased his forehead, and he said:

"I want to know what drugs can take the life of an athlete like Len Bias." Any psychoactive drug taken in high enough doses can cause death. Indeed, overdoses are the leading cause of death from drugs, but many other deaths are caused by complications from drug use:

Ethanol, the drug commonly called alcohol, is responsible for causing most adolescent deaths in the United States, from complications arising from its use such as murders, traffic accidents, falls, drownings, and fires.

1

Steve Prefontaine, one of America's greatest distance runners, died at the wheel of his sports car after drinking too much.

Heroin can cause death from AIDS and other viruses and bacteria when it is injected with contaminated needles.

Cocaine, abused for several weeks, can weaken the heart and cause death from cocaine-related cardiomyopathy.

Sensory blockers such as *PCP* can dull your senses so much that you could freeze to death or die from an injury you were unable to feel.

LSD causes hallucinations such as believing you have the ability to fly, and complications include death from falls.

Marijuana causes loss of coordination and memory and thus can cause reckless driving and fatal accidents.

Steroids used during hard training can cause fatal fluid loss. Birgit Dressel, German heptathlete, died in 1987, reportedly of a combination of painkillers and performance enhancers.

Beta blockers cause athletes to choke to death as airways to the lungs close in bronchospasm. They also can slow the heartbeat to the point of death.

Amphetamines cause blood vessels to narrow and change the heartbeat of an athlete who pushes too hard, causing death. Several world-class cyclists have died from use of amphetamines in their efforts to win.

Aspirin, the most widely used drug in the world, taken with large doses of vitamin C can cause a toxic buildup. Taken with sulfa antibiotics, it can increase the effects of the medication so as to be a fatal overdose. Used by competitive runners to run more coolly, aspirin can cause death from heat exhaustion by masking thirst and fatigue and by increasing fluid loss.

Diuretics were banned in 1986 because they were used to help athletes lose weight to meet weight limitations. In

1980 the lightweight Mr. Universe died of a heart attack caused by use of diuretics. A Swedish bodybuilder died from complications a few weeks later.

Cigarettes, both tobacco and marijuana, cause death from falling asleep while smoking and inhaling smoke from the resulting fire. Both types contain hundreds of toxic chemicals and cause long-term deaths from emphysema, cancer, and heart disease.

Chewing tobacco and *snuff* cause deaths from mouth cancer. Track athlete Sean Marsee died such a death at the age of nineteen.

Successful performance in sports depends upon having quick chemical reactions in your brain and a responsive muscle system that is efficient in directing such abilities as speed of movement, reaction time, agility, flexibility, and coordination. If you are good at sports it is because your nerves and muscles make fast and effective connections throughout your brain and body.

Drugs interfere with and replace the brain's normal processes during adolescent development. Some drugs such as marijuana affect the mind by reducing motivation. Too much marijuana can make you lose the "get up and go" feeling you need to train for sports so that you are no longer capable of doing your personal best.

Most athletes who use drugs do not die, but many fail at their sport. Here, using fictitious names, are some examples of how they fail:

Marijuana: Andy's depth perception is off. He can no longer judge the distance of the basket, or his team members, or the opponents. He looks as if he is moving in slow motion, and his timing is poor. He can't recall the strategies he knew so well because his memory fails to function. But his performance is hurt most by painful and disturbing muscle spasms, and he has to quit. The drug makes him lose his will to try, to finish, or to continue training. It makes him easily frustrated; he no longer cares, and he quits the team. Andy no longer wants to associate with the team members or any of his athlete friends.

Cocaine: What a hotshot Barry thinks he is. Suddenly he knows the secret of instant world-class stardom. He does not bother with training any more. Because of cocaine, he thinks he knows things that he doesn't and can do things for which he is unprepared. He is going to show up the competition because, in his paranoia, he thinks they are all out to make a fool of him. He is going to compete in events for which he has not trained. He enters the hurdles race and injures himself seriously because he competes beyond his ability.

Amphetamines: Charley's basketball playing becomes confused because of lack of rest and shortened rapid eye movement (REM) dreaming during sleep. He keeps hearing things that nobody said and seeing plays that didn't happen. His performance is also disturbed by his rapid, uneven heartbeat. He does not realize that he is hallucinating.

Nicotine: Tobacco smoking has really worn Don down. His resistance to disease is lowered, and he seems to get sick from everything going around. He has trouble sleeping, and he never was like that before. He can't train very long, and he needs more oxygen when he exercises. He thought he would quit smoking before his senior year, but he hasn't been able to do so.

Caffeine: Ed is having caffeine-induced anxiety attacks. He worries about little things. The drug is turning him into a hypochondriac, making him think things are wrong with his body. He has headaches when he goes without his caffeine pill or can't get a cup of strong coffee. He can't sleep, and sometimes he feels restless, irritable, and depressed about his whole life.

Beta blockers: Fred has a history of asthma, and he gets frightening bronchospasms that make him feel weak from the decrease in his blood pressure and the slowing of his heart. He has really weird dreams at night. His stomach gets upset, and he is losing a lot of hair. During competition he collapses, unable to breathe easily. He is rushed to the hospital, where the doctor says he will have to be admitted so they can get his breathing back to normal and slowly wean him from the drug.

Alcohol: George cannot aim well or move properly. His balance is not good, his reaction time is slow, and his hand-eye coordination is getting worse and worse. He comes close to being injured too often. He thought his muscle strength and endurance would improve, but instead he is losing weight because he has no appetite. His thinking is not what it used to be. His moods go from wild to violent, and he feels cold when he goes outside. He thinks he needs another drink to warm himself, or to loosen up and relax, or to feel confident of his abilities again, but he's really losing it.

Barbiturates: Harry thinks he has what it takes to be great, but the reality is that he has never played worse. Sometimes he looks drunk and can't even walk, but he still feels on top of things. He can't understand why the coach is making him sit the game out.

Benzodiazepines: The stress of training seems too much for Izzy to handle, so he pops one more benny. He feels hung over and can't get his body to perform well. His muscles are weak, and he feels nauseated. Because the bennies have been keeping him from stage-four sleep, he feels worried. When he tries to quit he goes into convulsions, shakes and sweats, throws up, and has muscle cramps.

Skeletal muscle relaxants: John becomes nervous when putting for a golf championship, but the pills depress his central nervous system and he has less control than ever.

Analgesics: Because of an aching body, Kirk uses too much aspirin to keep up with football practice. The excess causes allergic responses, nausea, vomiting, headache with ringing in the ears, and bleeding. Kirk loses even more practice time.

Narcotic analgesics: Larry wants to continue playing football in spite of an old injury. He keeps taking the painkiller, more each time. He is preventing the injury from healing, becoming dependent on the drug, and flirting with death. He first got the drug from his doctor to relieve the inflammation in his knee, but the side effects are ruining his performance.

Ibuprofen: Matt accepted the drug to reduce the inflamation in his ankle and make the pain bearable enough for him to play soccer, but he is getting headaches, dizzy spells, and an upset stomach. If he is allergic to it he will have bronchial spasms. He is lucky to have a reaction that will help to keep him from playing until his injury has healed.

An athlete can also fail by dropping out of sports or by being kicked out either for poor performance or as punishment for illegal use of drugs.

Sports performance requires the most complicated physical movements. To be successful in those movements, the athlete's brain must be in excellent condition for receiving and sending messages that involve strategy, control, balance, agility, refinement of movement, and coordination along with an instant memory of what works. Those processes are negotiated by chemicals in the brain.

The chemicals are effective because they are the nutrients in the foods of our ancestors. From birth until death, your life will be influenced by your body's unique chemical reactions. What you do to strengthen or weaken what you have now will have a strong impact on your future. As an athlete, you want to attain your personal best. You would like to improve your sports performance to the maximum. As an adolescent, you are motivated to fulfill certain inner drives that will transform childhood dependencies into adult self-reliance.

You have a special growth force in your mind that will influence you to develop throughout your life. The force will guide you toward personal fulfillment through whatever career path you take. The role models who have guided you through childhood become part of the lessons your inner self has to draw upon for strength. But from now on you will be acting more and more from your own motives. You will need to know what will happen to yourself and others because of your actions. You will either pay the penalties for wrong decisions or gain the benefits of right ones.

Remember that drugs interfere with the natural chemical processes that affect your moods, behavior style, body movements, health and appearance, motivation to practice, memory, abilities, and the quality of everything you do. You will fail to get along, you will fail to be dependable, and your performance at sports will make you accident-prone, sickly, anxious and depressed, irritable and suspicious.

For any of those reasons you can feel so uncomfortable

that you drop out or be so hard to get along with that you are kicked out. Getting kicked out of sports because you failed to make good grades will be only part of the reason. You will not have done your training, showed up on time, or worked hard at sports, and the poor quality of your performance will be a source of embarrassment to you, your school, your teammates, and your community.

The information and suggestions given in this book are based on current findings. They can serve as a foundation for developing a real competitive edge based on the facts, not on drug-inflated fantasies of power.

CHAPTER 2

You Need Your Brain

for Sports

The coach asked, "What else do you want to know about sports and drugs?"

The young athlete answered right away: "I really want to know what drugs do to my body."

The coach answered with a grin, "You seem to have a strong interest in sports physiology; maybe you would be interested in a career like mine. You have good athletic ability, and your teammates like you. Sports physiology is part of biological science. Biologists teach us about the life processes, activities, and functions of an athlete's body. Knowing more about sports physiology will also help you train effectively."

Most of what is known about the brain has been learned recently. We have imaging machines that create computer graphics by monitoring the brain's electrochemical actions. Imaging machines can show which areas work harder to process drugs.

Many electrochemical actions take place when you

move. Your body and brain are a complex maze that includes your neuromuscular system. That very compact system has evolved over three million years so that it can function independently of conscious awareness and with awareness too. High-powered technology helps neuro-scientists study the system.

Your neuromuscular system "runs" on electrochemical energy, which comes from a well-balanced diet. The neuromuscular system sets up, relays, and adjusts sport signals between your brain and your fast-twitch and slow-twitch muscle fibers. Muscle performance depends on the type of fiber used.

Sports movement cannot happen unless the neuro-muscular system has been trained by practice and experi-ence. In your body, an electrical transfer of chemicals made from food and water has to follow trained nerve pathways. You cannot expect to become a good athlete just by eating well or by putting drugs in your body. You need to train those pathways with practice. Eating wisely and drinking plenty of water keeps the nerve pathways fueled for action.

The more biologists study the brain, the more complex they find it to be. In fact, the human neuromuscular system is more complicated than anything else in the known universe. It is more complicated than all the high technology humanity has created.

People use only about one percent of their brain capacity. Sports physiology is developing ways to increase that percentage to improve performance. Sports medicine, training, and analysis of the mechanics of movement are enabling athletes to learn techniques that will give them the advantage over competitors known as the "competitive edge."

Drugs that affect brain function are called psychoactive

drugs. All the drugs discussed in this book interfere with the brain's neuromuscular activities, functions, and processes. They do not interfere with only one area, however; they disrupt many areas at the same time.

Psychoactive drugs affect sports performance through the neuromuscular system, which relays signals between brain and body. All psychoactive drugs interfere with the natural fueling of energy processes. Drugs rob the neuromuscular system of essential nutrients.

To get back to normal after using drugs, you need to replace the particular vitamins and minerals the drugs have wasted. You can get back to normal only if you have not done too much damage.

Every part of your body has muscles that spread in various directions from your bones. They are called *skeletal muscles* and are attached to the bones by *tendons*.

To make the muscles move, they are sprayed with a chemical called *acetylcholine*. Acetylcholine is made from choline, which comes from eggs and other foods. Many psychoactive drugs interfere with acetylcholine.

Each skeletal muscle is built up of millions of cells. The tough cells on the outside are called *membrane*. Membrane is wrapped around a bundle of living fibers that are composed of long strands of muscle cells.

Sports movements are made by very complicated electrochemical and neuromuscular systems that work together. The system is trained by your practice or training. It reacts by sending signals to and from the brain. The signals are chemicals sent by electrical energy back and forth along the nerve pathways.

All over the muscle membrane are thousands of nerve cells called *neurons*. Each neuron branches in all directions into *dendrites*, a word that comes from the Greek word for "tree." A dendrite looks like a ball with branches spreading over the muscle membrane. The branching fibers grow like smaller and smaller twigs on the branch of a tree.

The neurons are what make the muscles move. They are called efferent or motor neurons. The twig-like extensions of the dendrites are called *dendritic spines*. There are about forty to one hundred spines on every cell. Each one receives information from other nerve cells.

The cell body puts together in one message the information it has received from neighboring cells. That message is sent to the next cell on the *axon chain*. The axon chain is the longest branch extending from the neuron; it connects with sensory nerves and motor axons.

Very fine, controlled sports movements use stretch receptors, called neuromuscular spindles, on the skeletal muscles. They regulate muscle tone and control the precise movements needed for the competitive edge in sports.

The nerve impulse is an electrical impulse carried by charged particles called *ions*. Ions are made of the nutrients potassium and sodium (salts).

Two nerve cells communicate with an impulse spark. The spark squirts neurotransmitter fluid with special chemical shapes from one nerve cell to another. The space between nerve cells is called a *synapse*. Sometimes more than one chemical shape can be transmitted across a synapse.

Motor nerves activate muscle movement and can receive up to thirty thousand transmissions. The electrical impulse squirts *acetylcholine*. That causes sodium to enter the muscle cell and make it contract (tighten) or relax, depending on the amount of sodium it receives.

All these parts of your neuromuscular system need to be nourished with water and a well-balanced diet of nutritious foods. If you take in drugs and junk foods your neuro-muscular system will work hard to heal you, but you will be handicapping or killing yourself by your careless choices. Drugs, including alcohol and cigarettes, interfere with every cell in your body.

Your neuromuscular system is different from everyone else's because of your drug and diet choices, other life-style choices or habits, your training, and your genes.

Each *gene* you have inherited from your ancestors defines your potential for physical functioning. Each gene is responsible for the enzymes that cause molecular reactions in neuroreceptors in your brain.

Your brain is basically like other brains, but yours has a unique combination of advantages and disadvantages. Drugs can destroy your inborn potential by affecting your brain. Drugs can be more harmful to you than to someone else if you have a genetic weakness.

Each person needs to make the most of strengths and try to compensate for weaknesses. Choosing the right sport for your combination of strengths and weaknesses can make the difference between being a flop or becoming a champion.

Many parts of the brain must work together, all at the same time, for sports performance. In the cerebral cortical area of your brain, electrical activity takes place at the same time as muscle movements. Without that area you could not move. You have probably seen what being drunk from alcohol does to movement.

A single brain neuron can be involved in coordinating movement by directing many muscles at once. The brain analyzes what is happening outside the body, anticipates what will happen, and tells the body how to move.

The brain functions by passing tiny chemical substances from one cell or neuron to another. The chemical substances, called *neurotransmitters*, are made from our food and water. When they are the right ones, they fit into receptors and the information is used to benefit the athlete's performance. The wrong substances (as from psychoactive drugs) do not fit the receptors exactly. The extra molecules cause all kinds of interference with actions. The interference not only damages balance, coordination, and precision of movement but affects many other processes and functions that contribute to performance.

Sensory information, such as what is seen or heard, becomes confused. The athlete responds in the wrong way. The mood of the athlete can be changed so that reactions are too slow or otherwise inappropriate. The increased tension can put stress into movements that should flow from a relaxed body for accuracy.

Each athlete has billions of billions of brain cells. Each brain cell can make thousands of connections for receiving and sending information. The brain sends signals. It puts the signals together from the neurotransmitters it receives from the neurons. At the end of the axons, the electrical impulse fires the neurotransmitters to a nearby dendrite. Axon branches can end at muscle fibers in a knob called the terminal bouton or button, which connects with sensory nerves and motor axons.

Axons connect brain and body in bundles of nerves that are sheltered in the *spinal cord*. Special cells exist in sense organs, muscles, skin, and even joints. They send neurotransmitters to the brain through sensory neurons in the spinal cord. The processing of information goes on in both directions. Brain and body respond to the neurotransmitters being sent both ways at the same time. All messages are sent through the spinal cord.

Your brain reacts to experiences by making new connections with what you have learned. Then the brain devises new ways to solve problems. Drugs interfere with the ability to solve problems.

Interneurons in your brain and spinal cord pick up nerve chemical messages and relay them to motor neurons. Motor neuron axons are spread out along grooves in the muscle fibers. They send out neurotransmitters that trigger the muscle action.

Many transmissions are needed to perform one single movement. *Proprioceptors* in the joints send chemical shapes (molecular structures) to the brain that let it know where the legs, arms, and other joints are located.

Some drugs, like alcohol, get into every cell in the body. Taking a drug that interferes with proprioceptors is like disconnecting the wires that make a robot move. An alcohol user loses proprioceptor efficiency and has trouble moving.

Opioids are chemical structures that fit exactly, "hand in glove," into areas of the brain called *opiate receptor sites*. Opioids are like rewards for being good to your body by satisfying its needs. Movement with rhythm, such as many sports movements have, causes your brain to release opioids such as *endorphins* and *enkephalins*. Opioids stimulate a desire for drinking water to quench thirst or eating food to satisfy hunger. They also help athletes take painful injuries in stride.

Psychoactive drugs can fill the opiate receptors and activate the reward feelings for hunger and thirst or pain and depression. The drugs make the athlete insensitive to those needs; he or she may be harmed greatly by the inhibition of these natural incentives for self-care.

Psychoactive drugs do not fit the opiate receptors cleanly. They stick out with additional chemical structures that trigger other reactions called side effects that include various forms of death and disease.

Experience and training build efficient networks in the brain and body for good performance. Drugs can destroy what all those workouts have created.

Once you appreciate the importance of choosing carefully what you put into your body, you can begin to take control of the actions that lead to successful sports performance. You can make decisions using standards that have been measured and tested and proven to work.

Biologists, especially neuroscientists, have discovered many ways in which the brain controls and develops sports performance. All movements, all actions and reactions are controlled by your brain. Everything you experience becomes part of you, and the results of what you learn stay in your brain and actually shape it. Training becomes inner paths to your best performance. Choosing a nutrient-loaded and balanced diet of natural foods will improve your performance.

Your brain cannot be overloaded with information. The smallest unit of information is called a *bit*. The brain can process a lot of bits of information at once. Millions of cells can be active at the same time.

Your reactions can be almost instantaneous (especially to pain). Brain neurons communicate instantly with neurotransmitters. Anything the body does, or any thought the brain thinks, makes the brain create and send out neurotransmitters. There are thirty known specific types of neurotransmitters.

Your brain is what keeps you alive. It makes your heart beat, your blood flow. It causes your food to be broken down into usable chemicals. It gives you dreams, thoughts, feelings, and solutions to problems.

Sights and sounds are used as cues to guide your movements. Your body temperature is controlled by your brain, even while you sleep. Your survival skills improve every night while you sleep. Your brain has noticed more details than your waking mind could be aware of. Waking awareness is only part of what the brain learns each day. The brain solves problems during sleep at night, especially when they are goal-oriented problems as for doing better at a sport.

Your brain fights disease. It directs your *immune system* by sending out *macrophages*, large white blood cells, to fight disease organisms such as viruses or bacteria. The immune system mends and strengthens torn muscle tissues after you have given them moderate stress by training. It makes you stronger for the next workout.

Emotions and feelings are also controlled by your brain. Drugs damage the neurotransmitters in the brain known as *biogenic amines*. The biogenic amines are subdivided into the *catecholamines*: epinephrine, dopamine, and norepinephrine (noradrenaline), and the *indoleamines*: tryptophan and serotonin.

If too few of the biogenic amines are sent through your brain, you feel depressed and sad, not very hungry, and have trouble concentrating and sleeping. Your muscle tension and heart and breathing rates increase, and your nervous system has an imbalance of electrical charges from too much salt and too much of the hormone *cortisol*.

You need extra nutrients while your hormones are making you grow. If you use drugs, you rob your body of necessary nutrients such as vitamins, minerals, proteins, and amino acids, especially the biogenic amines.

Drugs burn the fuels needed by the neuromuscular system. The nutrients wasted by drug use need to be replaced before you can train well again. An athlete cannot perform at peak level when taking any drug.

Drugs that lower serotonin levels in the brain cause aggression. Low levels of serotinin can be caused by lack of enough good carbohydrates in your body. As an athlete, you need to make sure your energy output is fueled with adequate carbohydrates. Carbohydrates are obtained from whole grains, which are usually less expensive than other foods and can be eaten in large amounts by athletes without doing harm. The nutrients in whole grains are important for growth processes.

The neurotransmitter acetylcholine is essential to memory. People whose brain lacks enough acetylcholine suffer from forgetfulness and have difficulty learning. Acetylcholine assists in unlocking the hormone *vasopressin* in the brain; it thus starts the *action potential* in your muscles. The action potential spreads through muscle, making it contract so that you can move.

It is foolish to expect the wrong fuels—drugs—to outperform the right fuels—foods. Brain function and sports performance improve with good foods and drug avoidance.

CHAPTER 3

Risks, Penalties
and Injuries

The laws of physiology, of your own body, are more apt to sentence you to capital punishment (death) than to penalties for a positive drug test. Think about it.

Nobody can take your training away from you. But drugs can ruin what it has taken you a lifetime to develop. All potential can be lost when your body and mind are damaged by drugs.

In the nature of chemical reactions, what hurts one neuromuscular system may not hurt another. Because there are so many effects, the risks are high for everyone.

Each person's body has slightly different chemical reactions. It depends upon genetic heritage, diet, and stress levels. Your body and mind cannot be replaced like worn-out sports equipment. Medical therapy can be very expensive once health is lost, and the effort usually cannot be made without professional counseling, which is also expensive. Some athletes take better care of their uniforms and sports equipment than of their bodies.

To develop into adults, teenagers need to explore and even take calculated (meaning probably safe) risks. Exploring ideas and feelings, drives and ambitions is enough to develop an independent adult self. It can feel risky to discuss your deepest self, your fears and dreams.

Professor Neil D. Weinstein of Rutgers University wrote an article* about the risk factor as seen by adults and teenagers. He found that most adults are apt to think of themselves as protected against personal risks such as drug addiction and disease, when in fact they are at risk. Each adult tends to think his chances of success and long life are greater than those of other people.

He found that few people who engaged in high-risk sexual behavior or drug use thought of their own risk as being high. They believed that having only a few sex partners, or not seeing signs of AIDS on their partner, or even taking a shower after sex could keep them safe. That is definitely not true.

Teenagers have always felt less vulnerable, less likely to be harmed, than any other group. Many high school students who thought they could drink or smoke marijuana and drive are now dead. Others who rode with them are dead too. Many graduation parties are drug-free these days to prevent such tragedies.

According to Professor Weinstein, "Reasoning is distorted to yield self-serving predictions." In other words, adults want to do well so they think they can get by with risky behaviors because of some other trait.

For instance, a strong healthy looking athlete will look in the mirror and find it hard to believe that an invisible virus

* *Science*, Vol. 246, p. 1232.

or a drug could kill such a body. But they can and do kill.

Healthy, athletic teenagers can learn the reality of risky behaviors. Personal harm, including death, can come from using drugs. When teenagers are informed of the dangers, they can become more self-protective than most adults.

Many of the deaths from drugs are going to be from AIDS. People who contract AIDS will die because there is no cure. By the year 2000 a vaccine may be available, but for many that will be too late.

Because of illegal drug use, including alcohol, more American teenagers than ever before are becoming involved in sexual activity. The risks are greater than ever.

Drug addicts tell lies, even in marriages, about sexual relationships with other people. An infected person can look and feel healthy for several years before symptoms of AIDS appear.

The time has come for American students to help everyone face the risks and become better protected. Athletes can set a good example. The first step is to learn the dangers.

Alcohol, amphetamines, amyl nitrite, marijuana, and cocaine are drugs that block the part of the brain that exercises good judgment. You might make a bad decision that causes you to lose a game. You might become suddenly violent because those drugs also shut off the part of the brain that controls aggressive behavior.

Drugs alter behavior in many ways. They cause unpredictable outbursts and actions beyond your control. They can cause aggressive acts of violence, and even murder. The violence of gang wars is often inflated by members under the influence of drugs such as alcohol, steroids, PCP, and amphetamines. Random and even acquaintance rape is sometimes precipitated by the use of alcohol and/or drugs.

Teens are notorious risk takers. Dangerous behavior can

result when under the influence of alcohol and drugs. Your judgment and the decisions you make can be seriously impaired by drugs. It is frequently life-threatening.

The use of crack cocaine has been cited for the increase in unsafe sex practices that lead to sexually transmitted diseases (STDs) and acquired immunodeficiency syndrome (AIDs). Teens are at risk for AIDS when using unclean needles and engaging in unprotected sex.

The Centers for Disease Control (CDC) also reports that females have been contracting AIDS from sharing intravenous (IV) needles and syringes contaminated with blood containing the HIV virus. Risky behavior even "just once" can allow the virus to enter your body. There is no cure.

GROWTH RATES

Drugs cause poor judgment. In sports they dramatically increase your chances of being injured. Playing sports while you are still growing is risk enough. From the ages of eleven to eighteen teenagers go through very stressful physical and mental changes. Each athlete develops adult form during those years. Learn about the changes, then decide how you can cope with them.

Physical growth rates can vary widely. Your personal growth rate is one factor that determines how vulnerable to injury you are and how sensitive to pain. Drugs will affect you differently at each stage of your growth. Your increasing size will affect your ability to process drugs.

Only after your skeleton has reached full size can your muscles fill out and become able to use oxygen for energy efficiently.

In boys there can be a five-year lag in starting to develop a larger skeleton. Boys may take two years longer than girls just for their legs to grow. During that growth period boys need to protect themselves from injury to the long-bone growth plates. Such injury can stop growth and cripple a boy for life.

CONTACT SPORTS

Rough contact sports like wrestling, football, hockey, and lacrosse can put you in a position to be hit hard in a growth plate. Do not play when injured, in pain, on drugs, or against players on drugs who may become too aggressive. To avoid the risk of injury, be careful to play sports with opponents of your size and level of experience.

Only boys whose feet have not grown for eighteen months should play rough contact sports. When the feet stop growing the skeleton has reached its full growth. During a year and a half after that the bones and muscles become solid and strong. The upper body also develops during that time.

It takes extra nutriment and extra rest to accomplish all that growth. Take it easy when you feel tired. Drink plenty of nourishing fluids. Reduce your risk of injury by paying attention to your changing needs.

PAIN

Sports training can increase your production of *endorphins*, the natural painkillers, and protect you from feeling too much pain. You need to receive some pain as a warning that your body needs care when overstressed or harmed. The purpose of pain is to make you rest so that your immune system can heal the stress or injury. You need to pay attention to it.

You risk injury in any sport. You can easily sprain

ligaments or strain muscles. Be careful while your tendons, ligaments, and skeleton are still growing. Some injuries could cause trouble the rest of your life.

Overuse of your body while you are growing fast can also cause problems. Until your growth slows, take it easy. Usually you will not feel like pushing during the fast-growth period. If you overdo, you can get small bone cracks (stress fractures), which also cause pain from shin splints. Follow a doctor's directions to heal them.

These injuries are caused by gradual wear and tear without enough rest for repairs. Using drugs can interfere with getting enough rest. Injuries can result from concentrating on one sport for too long. Running and tennis injuries are mostly from overuse. Not building up other muscle systems can also make you vulnerable to injury. Runners sometimes neglect to develop their upper bodies enough to strengthen them against injury.

When you are tired, you put greater strain on your body by not moving correctly. Giving yourself rest can be more important than "pushing through the pain."

Switching to a different sport too quickly can also cause pain from shin splints (in the front of your leg between ankle and knee). Always make changes gradually in training and competitive performance. Drugs sometimes make athletes feel powerful enough to handle athletic events for which they are not trained, so they are at greater risk of injury.

Pain should be managed according to its cause. A teenage athlete suffering from overuse pain should slow down. An athlete who has pain from straining skeletal muscles should rest until healed, then build up gradually.

Pain usually feels like the problem, but it is not; it is merely a good clue to help diagnose an injury. Masking pain with a drug does nothing to cure an injury, unless it is used to help you sleep when the pain interferes with your rest. Pain is a useful signal for treating an injury. If the signal is turned off, you feel you can use the injured muscle, tendon, ligament, or other part. If you do so, you risk making the injury much worse or even incurring a new injury. Drugs can also cause excitement and determination, which can keep you from feeling pain.

Painkillers are *adjunctive therapies*, which means that they are not as important as the treatment of the injury. You need to be very careful not to use the injured area except as your doctor recommends. Taking even a few weeks off to heal completely is very important. It can protect you from permanent or prolonged injury.

Learn first aid for sports injuries. Be careful not to use the injured part if the pain is severe. Applying ice or pressure or both on trigger points (tender muscle knots caused by stress and injury) may help. You can also learn to use your mind to slow down and even stop the pain signals with endorphins.

PAINKILLERS

Tell your coach and doctor when you experience pain. They can help you find out what causes it. Only your doctor should prescribe or give you drugs for pain. Your doctor should first carefully evaluate and treat the cause of the pain.

With painkillers, as with any prescription, let your doctor and pharmacist know that you are an athlete. You want them to know you need to protect your central nervous system by avoiding depressant drugs that mask but do not cure pain. Remind them that you do not want to be able to forget and use the injured part and thus damage it even more. As an athlete, it is your responsibility to protect yourself from painkillers that could hurt your performance in any way.

Nonnarcotic painkillers are useful when combined with healing efforts aimed at the injury. If pain keeps you awake, a painkiller can help you rest so that your body can repair itself.

You experience pain when the stressed, threatened, or injured area sends chemicals to the *thalamus* of the brain, where it is detected. The thalamus sends electrochemical messages to the cortex, which decodes them and develops a response. When your calf aches you rub it and endorphins are released, making you feel better. *Opioids* (endorphins and enkephalins) are released to help you survive under life-threatening circumstances too. They are released along with the pain to enable you to cope with it in a useful way.

The easiest pain to locate is from skin injuries. Called *cutaneous*, meaning "affecting the skin," it is also known as "fast pain" because it is transmitted easily through thick fibers. It feels sharp, burning, or prickly and does not last very long. You can usually figure out quickly what caused it.

Athletes tend to have problems with *deep pain*, caused by stressing or injuring muscles, tendons, joints, or bones. The ache tends to last. It can be hard to define because it may seem to be coming from a nearby area as *referred* pain.

The internal organs also create referred pain because they do not have nerve endings that act as pain receptors. It is called *visceral* pain. Visceral and deep pain are called *slow pain* because it travels slowly through thin fibers.

Drugs can create pain or block it or both. Pain receptors are acted upon by drugs. Whenever the brain is under stress it becomes chemically imbalanced and can produce pain.

Pain enhancers and painkillers are both found in the same area of the brain. The pain-control area is called the *rostial ventromedial medulla*. It has two sets of nerve cells, "on cells" and "off cells," which regulate the experience of pain by increasing it or blocking it.

Pain chemicals called *prostaglandins* are made by cells near the injured cells. Aspirin blocks prostaglandin release.

CHAPTER 4

Self-Defense Techniques for Legal Drugs

Prescription drugs are intended to be used only with a doctor's permission and only by the person for whom they were prescribed. Prescription drugs injure and kill three times as many people as heroin every year. There are many reasons why they are so harmful.

Prescriptions must be written based on a careful evaluation of need. A qualified and ethical doctor needs to decide from your symptoms what is wrong with you. Even a well-trained doctor can make the wrong evaluation sometimes.

The doctor should consider your personal chemistry. He or she should know about any bad reactions you may have had. Other drugs, foods, and food supplements can interact with medications. Your age and size can make a difference between giving too much of a drug, which could injure you, or too little, which might not cure you. The doctor decides on the most effective dose at the time the prescription is written.

Your personal chemistry changes as you grow, so prescription refills can be dangerous if made too long after being prescribed. Some drugs need to be monitored to be sure you continue to get the right amount.

Prescription drugs are most harmful when they are taken by people for whom they were not prescribed. No one should take another person's prescription medicine. Even if the symptoms, age, and weight seem the same, the cause of the symptoms and personal reactions can be drastically different.

There are many reasons for avoiding drugs while you are still growing. Most drugs are designed for adults. Drugs applied to the skin (like dimethyl sulfoxide, DMSO) are called *topical*. Until you are fully grown your skin is thin and will absorb more of the drug than adult skin.

While you are young, you also have more fluid in your body weight than you will have as an adult. Drugs that dissolve in water will spread to more places in your body than in an adult's. They move through fluids to their receptors.

As you get older you have more fat in your body. Drugs that dissolve in fats will not spread as easily as in adults but will remain more concentrated, with stronger effects.

Some drugs are metabolized faster in children than in adults, so children need higher doses for effective treatment.

Your weight and the measurement of the surface area of your body are also considerations in prescribing drugs.

The use of drugs has been accepted by doctors for crisis situations in which the benefits are greater than the risks and side effects. When you take any medication you should try to understand why the benefits outweigh the risks. Soon we may have medicines without side effects, possibly by using food substances for healing.

The people who make our medicines follow definite rules and precise measurements. New medicines are first tested in the laboratory and perhaps on animals. Then they are tested on a small group of people, who are watched very carefully for side effects. The small group is called a *control group*. Finally the drug is described in scientific terms to detail everything that has been observed about its effects on the control group. Then it must be approved by the Food and Drug Administration before it can be dispensed to the public.

Since the late 1980s some doctors have been selling drugs themselves, to increase their incomes. Beware of such practices. Double-check with a pharmacist. Some doctors are themselves addicted to drugs. Some are very careless in writing prescriptions. A decimal point in the wrong place can mean getting the wrong dose.

Sometimes doctors prescribe drugs that are banned by athletic associations and the International Olympic Committee (IOC). It is the responsibility of the athlete to learn the rules and follow them. The standards are set for the safety of the athlete.

Athletes should find out whether a prescribed drug will cause potassium or sodium (electrolyte) loss. Long workouts cause fluid loss, which can cause electrolyte imbalance.

Know how to store your medicines. Some drugs need refrigeration; others need to be protected from warmth, moisture, or light. Poor environmental conditions can lead to drug failure or harm because of chemical changes.

Discard medicine that has passed its expiration date. The chemistry can be quite different than when it was fresh.

Black market prescription drugs are sold (illegally) for profit. They are more likely to be old, exposed to the wrong conditions, and thus changed chemically.

Be very careful to reach for the right medicine. People have been injured or killed from taking the wrong medicine. Labels and containers can look very much alike but be very different. The illegal market for prescription drugs is especially apt to sell "look-alikes" (counterfeit drugs). Remember, the wrong drug can kill you. Do not accept drugs from "friends." No matter how much you like them, they may be using you to earn money.

Ask your pharmacist for an information sheet about your prescription medicine. It will explain what it can do to help, the correct way to take it, and potential dangers of the drug. Drug failure is sometimes caused by taking foods or other drugs at the same time, which can change the chemistry of the drug or block it. The information sheet will also warn you of possible dangerous side effects.

If you have a bad reaction, seek advice right away. Call an emergency clinic, a pharmacist, or your doctor.

Remember that any drug affects many areas of your neuromuscular system. The needed effects of the drug make it worthwhile for you to take it only if the risk from side effects is not too great.

People have a wide range of reactions to drugs. Read the information sheet to know which side effects are within the expected range and which are dangerous.

Many teenagers are careless about medications. Some forget to take them, some take too much at a time or take them at the wrong times. Many stop taking medication too soon, with the result that the illness, perhaps infectious to others, is not cured.

It is estimated that about half of the many millions of prescriptions written for teenagers are not taken as directed. It is very important to take medicine exactly as the doctor prescribed.

Some teenagers think that if one pill is good, two must be twice as good. That can cause a drug overdose. Just a few extra spoonfuls of the tasty cough syrup might land you in the emergency room. Alcohol, codeine, and other ingredients sometimes found in cough syrup could make you feel and be worse off than you would have been without it. Alcohol and codeine can lead to addiction. There are nonaddictive drugs for every medicinal need; do not accept addictive drugs.

In spite of all the checks and balances of the American drug regulation process, problems occur. Read the labels and know what is in medicines before taking them. Some work best when taken on an empty stomach, others work best with milk or a meal. Many react with other medicines, foods, or drinks. They can cause every reaction from bad feelings to death.

To protect yourself, tell your doctor that you do not want anything addictive. Ask the pharmacist, when you fill the prescription, if there is anything addictive in it. If there is, the doctor can be called to change the medication to a nonaddictive one that the pharmacist can recommend.

Doctors may not know about the drug restrictions for amateur athletes. They may prescribe a banned substance that could make you test positive for drug abuse. It is your responsibility to learn which drugs to avoid.

How can you learn? Reading this book will give you an excellent start. You can always ask a pharmacist or librarian for help in making decisions about specific prescriptions. The United States Olympic Committee (USOC) hotline will help if you have questions about banned substances. The toll-free hotline telephone number is: 1/800/233–0393.

The USOC will also send you the current *Guide to Banned Medications*. The Guide states:

> Be especially alert to the exact name of your medication because many sound alike. For example, Tylenol and Afrin are acceptable medications to take. On the other hand Co-Tylenol and Afrinaol are banned medications. Chlor-Trimeton, a common antihistamine, is safe, but any combination of Chlor-Trimeton with a decongestant is banned. New products appear on the market almost monthly, so beware of this caution. This list is always subject to changes and will be revised and updated annually.

OVER-THE-COUNTER DRUGS

Lower doses of prescription drugs are often sold over-the-counter (OTC) along with safer drugs. Buyers and users are trusted to use OTC drugs according to the directions on the label and to watch for side effects.

You could take a banned substance that might eliminate you from competition when tested for drugs. It is your responsibility to learn what drugs to stay away from.

For instance, as an athlete you are responsible for learning how to medicate a cough while avoiding banned substances. If you cough up yellow to green colored mucus, you should see a doctor for diagnosis. You might have a lung infection.

If the mucus is clear, however, you can use a vaporizer or humidifier to moisten the air without needing medicine at all (unless you have an allergy).

When you cannot be in moist air, only one medicinal

ingredient will help you cough out more of the infected mucus. It is *quaifenesin*, the only expectorant approved by the Food and Drug Administration (FDA) as of February, 1990.

For a dry cough (without mucus) you can use a cough suppressant. Doctors still sometimes prescribe codeine, which—besides being addictive—can make you sleepy, upset your stomach, and make you constipated. For those reasons, the IOC recommends only nonnarcotic Dextromethorphan.

Cough and cold formulas can contain as many as seven drugs in combination. Called "shotgun" remedies, they usually contain an antihistamine, which does not even treat colds or coughs, but only allergic reactions. They often contain a decongestant that masks the symptoms and prevents you from coughing out infected mucus. Sometimes they also contain a pain reliever that can be harmful.

The risks of side effects increase whenever drugs are combined. You may be getting or creating within your body a new drug that your body cannot handle.

Even if you need medicine for aches and pains as well as a decongestant, the amounts of each in a cold formula may be the opposite of the effects you need. You may get too much of the decongestant, which can worsen your condition with a rebound effect. You may get too little of the pain reliever. Worse yet, you might get too much pain reliever and harm yourself.

Decongestants dry the mucus caused by colds and allergies. If you take them for more than a few days you can permanently damage your mucous membranes. Decongestants make some people feel lazy or even sleepy, spacy and irritable, restless, or unable to concentrate. A rebound effect when they wear off can make you feel even worse, because your ears and nose become clogged. Decongestants are often combined with aspirin or acetaminophen. Be careful; read and follow the directions.

Cough suppressants are depressants of the central nervous system. All such depressants interfere with thinking and organized muscle actions needed for sports. An athlete needs to think quickly and move efficiently to perform well.

Antihistamines are helpful for coughs and sneezes caused by allergies, but not for colds and other coughs. They are sometimes added to cold and cough formulas but do no good unless you are treating an allergy.

Benadryl Elixir is labeled as a "children's allergy medication," but it contains 14 percent alcohol, sugar, and red dyes as well as Benadryl. Those extra ingredients can cause problems. Benadryl itself is an IOC-allowable drug. Read labels carefully and talk with your pharmacist and doctor.

Tablets are usually a safer choice than liquid medicines because they do not contain alcohol. Look for "alcohol-free" liquid medications.

CAFFEINE

Cough and analgesic (pain-relieving) drugs often contain caffeine, which growing athletes need to avoid. It takes about eight hours for the body to metabolize caffeine. If you metabolize food quickly, caffeine can be more harmful to you. Caffeine interferes with fine muscle coordination.

Girls on birth control pills take up to sixteen hours to metabolize caffeine. Caffeine taken at noon with lunch could interfere with sleep until four the next morning. Caffeine is a mild stimulant, which means that it is psychoactive, affecting many areas of the brain. Caffeine can also worsen premenstrual syndrome (PMS) symptoms.

Caffeine in high doses is banned by the IOC. It is best not to make a habit of using it. With use, more and more caffeine is needed to get the same stimulant effect. Needing higher doses to get the same effect is called developing *tolerance.*

Caffeine tends to dull the appetite. Filling up on empty calories ("junk foods" without nutrients) can lead to nutritional deficit. Caffeine is often found in colas, hot chocolate, coffee, and tea. Candy bars, cakes, cookies, ice cream, and other foods may also contain caffeine.

Many people like the stimulant effect of caffeine to wake them up in the morning. Cold water wakes your brain better than a hot drink. Cold juice or milk also helps get you going without side effects.

Six hundred milligrams a day of caffeine or less for normal adolescents can interfere with sports performance by causing frequent urination, nervousness, anxiety, restlessness, paranoia, and tingling in fingers and toes. It can make it hard to get enough sleep because you will wake up more often during the night. Teenagers need nine and a half hours sleep every night just to grow. You need even more sleep when you train for sports. If you do not get enough, you stress your body and are more apt to injure yourself.

Caffeine also interferes with the ability to absorb iron, which is needed to make red blood cells. Iron is also part of many brain enzymes that energize the brain as neurotransmitters.

Caffeine wastes several important nutrients. Potassium, which is used during exercise, is wasted by caffeine. Potassium is contained in dried fruits, tomatoes, oranges, and roasted peanuts. Athletes need about 99 mg of potassium every day. With use of caffeine you need even more.

Caffeine wastes the body's supply of zinc, which is needed for normal growth, healing, and appetite. Caffeine wastes the body's supply of the vitamin biotin. Loss of biotin can cause loss of appetite, muscle pain, skin problems, anemia, and sleeplessness.

Caffeine interferes with the absorption and metabolism of thiamine (vitamin B_1). Thiamine is needed for metabolism of carbohydrates, which are required for energy.

Loss of calcium takes place 100 percent faster and magnesium 50 percent faster with just 300 mg of caffeine. Magnesium transmits nerve and muscle impulses; no athlete can function well without it. You need calcium for bone strength, muscle growth and contraction, and to prevent muscle cramps. Calcium also contributes fuel for energy.

Girls need extra calcium if they go out for sports. They lower their estrogen level by strenuous workouts. Estrogen helps calcium strengthen girls' bones.

Caffeine raises blood cholesterol levels. Cholesterol leaves fatty deposits on the walls of arteries, which can eventually close and cause death to heart and brain. Most cholesterol, 80 percent, is made in the liver. Caffeine is toxic to the liver.

Caffeine blocks adenosine receptors. *Adenosine* is a natural tranquilizer. Blocking it is what provides the stimulant effect. Do not forget the nervousness, anxiety, and restlessness effects that also go with it.

Caffeine wastes brain neurotransmitters such as *norepinephrine*, one of the biogenic amines. Norepinephrine is a transmitter that causes sensory arousal for quick response to danger. It helps to focus attention and awareness and improves memory and learning. It is also released and wasted by the use of other stimulant drugs such as amphetamines and cocaine. Norepinephrine fiber makes up only about 1 percent of the total transmitters in your brain, but it affects all parts of it. Foods containing amino acids are needed to replace it.

EPHEDRINE

Ephedrine, a stimulant banned by the IOC, does not improve performance. It has been one of the most difficult for athletes to protect themselves against. Ephedrine masks fatigue. It is an ingredient of "sports supplements" and "diet aids" and is often found in health food stores in its natural form. It is also contained in over-the-counter medications such as antihistamines or "shotgun" cold remedies.

"Natural herbal combinations" sound safe but they can be harmful when they include the natural form of ephedrine. They are sold under many names: Ma Huang, Brigham Tea, Bishop's Tea, Chi Powder, Energy Ris, Ephedra, Excel, Joint Fir, Mexican Tea, Miner's Tea, Mormon Tea, Popotillo, Squaw Tea, Super Charge, and Teamster's Tea. Drug testing for ephedrine readily picks up the herbal form because it mimics amphetamines, but it affects a different part of the brain. Golden Seal Tea is another stimulant sold in health food stores as a herbal tea.

ASTHMA REMEDIES

To relieve asthmatic swollen breathing passages, the IOC allows the use of a topical decongestant with the single active ingredient *oxymetazoline*. It is found in Afrin Nasal Spray, in Duration and Dristan Long-Lasting Nasal Spray, and in Vicks Sinex Long-Acting Nasal Spray.

Inhaled *corticosteroids* are safe for asthma conditions. They act only topically, meaning where they are applied.

They are sold as *beclomethasone, triamcinolone,* and *fluoniside*.

The yearly death rate from asthma has nearly doubled in ten years, from 2,500 to 4,000, probably from pollution and abuse of inhalants.

Besides bronchodilators, asthmatic athletes should use antiinflamatory drugs against secondary attacks, which happen as long as eight hours later, according to the National Institute of Allergy.

Intramuscular and intravenous corticosteroids mask pain from injuries, which puts the athlete in danger of reinjury. They can prevent healing and lead to an overgrowth of infection. Their use is banned by the USOC.

CHAPTER ◇ 5

Pain Relievers
and Painkillers

Nonsteroidal antiinflammatory drugs (NSAIDs) are sold over-the-counter and are widely advertised. They are used by athletes to reduce pain. Using NSAIDs and playing sports increases the risk of injury. They are not addictive, but they can become a dangerous habit.

In Chapter 2 we discussed sports injuries and pain. When you are injured, various types of *prostaglandins* are made by your cells to cope with the injury. They cause the area to become inflamed, causing swelling, heat, and pain.

Your blood contains tiny bodies called platelets. When a blood vessel is cut, platelets adhere to the membranes and plug them until blood clots form to stop the bleeding. Prostaglandins regulate platelet function and blood vessel tone.

Some NSAIDs lock into a type of protein molecule that blocks chemical structures that signal pain. High doses of the drugs control the rate at which red blood cells move through the plasma. They also alter the amount of C-reactive protein the liver makes to fight infection.

Natural pain enhancers and painkillers are both found in the same area of the brain, the rostial ventromedial medulla. The pain-modulating area has two sets of nerve cells, called "on-cells" and "off-cells" because they regulate the experience of pain. Increased sensitivity to pain is called *hyperalgesia*, a condition often caused in drug addicts during withdrawal.

ASPIRIN

The NSAID most abused in the United States is *aspirin*. Many dangerous reactions occur from its use. Every year more than 10,000 people develop salicylism from an overdose of aspirin. They become nauseated, vomit, and have headache and ringing in the ears. Some people die. Aspirin overdose can cause allergic responses and excessive bleeding after sports injuries. It can cause visual problems, thirst, excessively rapid breathing, called *hyperventilation*, and heart trouble. Aspirin is often mixed with the addictive drug *codeine* in cough and cold formulas.

Aspirin can be very dangerous to the growing body. In 1963 an Australian pediatrician, Douglas Reye (pronounced rye), described certain symptoms as part of an illness that is named for him, Reye's syndrome. Until then the symptoms had been ascribed to poisoning, drug overdose, meningitis, or encephalitis.

If you take aspirin for a virus infection, especially flu or chicken pox, you can get the terrible symptoms of Reye's syndrome. It causes uncontrollable vomiting, confusion, and swelling of the brain and liver. Without treatment, convulsions and coma may end in death.

OTHER NSAIDs

Researcher Gerald Weissmann studied the cells most often found in cases of acute inflammation, the *neutrophils*. In an article* he explained how NSAIDs interact with cell chemistry. He discovered that the drugs prevent neutrophils from sticking together and releasing enzymes, peptides, and irritants that damage tissues. Some NSAIDs were found to keep neutrophils from sticking to blood vessel walls. In the tissue injury processes, cells leave the circulatory system, causing inflammation. The NSAIDs change inflammatory cells in many ways. They also slow down bone metabolism and the making of cartilage. They act on the disease-fighting macrophages and on monocytes.

The NSAIDs are chemically unrelated drugs that can be divided into three main groups according to chemical structure: (1) four types of carbolic acid; (2) pyrazoles; and (3) oxicams. None of the categories is addictive, but taking them for pain can become a risky habit.

The main chemical danger from all NSAIDs is taking them too soon after a soft-tissue injury. They increase the bleeding into soft tissue.

Drug testing of athletes with enzyme immunoassay (EIA) and radioimmunoassay (RIA) techniques have given false positives because of NSAIDs such as *ibuprofen* and *naproxen*. Further testing can show the difference.

Acetaminophen, the ingredient in Tylenol and other OTC analgesics, is not useful as an antiinflammatory drug. It is mainly used as a pain reliever. Overdose can cause acetaminophen poisoning with symptoms such as pain, stomach cramps, diarrhea, nausea, and vomiting. Severe liver damage can be fatal in overdoses.

* *Scientific American*, January 1991.

Ibuprofen, another commonly used OTC ingredient, is found in Advil and Motrin and is similar to chemicals like naproxen and fenoprofen, which are prescription drugs. They interfere with blood clotting and upset the stomach. Ibuprofen should not be taken with caffeine.

Phenacetin is used to relieve pain and reduce fever. It is usually combined with aspirin and caffeine as APC. It is almost free of side effects if taken as directed for a limited time. Large doses cause poisoning. Eleven- to twelve-year-olds should not take it for more than five days, and adults should not take it for more than ten days, so adolescents need to be very careful.

Skeletal muscle relaxants (SMRs) are neuromuscular blockers. They depress the central nervous system and slow transmission of nerve impulses from the spinal cord to the skeletal muscles. Athletes who have pain caused by muscle contractions take an SMR to slow the contractions and reduce the pain.

The drugs also slow the reflexes. An athlete cannot respond as quickly or as accurately when taking an SMR. Muscle spasms occur because of inflammation. Icepacks are better first aid. The drugs are not useful for recovery, and the risks are too great for relief of short-lived pain.

SMRs cause feelings of dizziness, weakness, fatigue, and confusion, which are made worse by inability to sleep. They can cause seuzures. They increase heart tension and hyperglycemia and cause nausea, constipation, and urinary frequency.

Social life is apt to suffer because of skin rashes, swollen ankles, heavy sweating, and weight gain. Use with other depressants, including alcohol, intensifies the effects. Breathing can stop permanently. Sudden withdrawal from the drugs can cause hallucinations and spastic movements.

Dimethyl sulfoxide (DMSO) has been used to treat

skeletal muscle problems. DMSO is found in all plants. The main liquid in tree sap, it moves the nutrients from the roots to the trunk, branches, twigs, and leaves along long lines of cells.

Although much evidence of the benefits of DMSO as a drug has been reported since the 1960s, it is still not allowed for athletic uses. Industrial grade DMSO, a waste product of the lumber industry, is used illegally for tendinitis and bursitis. It is not of good enough quality for such use.

DMSO needs to be made under sterile, controlled conditions. Because of its carrier capability it can move dangerous chemicals quickly from cell to cell into the bloodstream and past the blood-brain barrier. Such dangerous chemicals could be on the skin or in the industrial grade DMSO.

DMSO is banned by the IOC. Its medical quality is now being researched for use by athletes with tendinitis and bursitis under sterile conditions by specially trained doctors. Even in its best form, it causes side effects of skin rash, nausea, and headaches.

NARCOTIC ANALGESICS

The word *narcotic* comes from the Greek word meaning "deadening." Deadening perfectly describes the effects of narcotic analgesics. They deaden the user's ability to recognize, by feeling pain, an injury; they thus deaden the user's ability to manage by taking care of the part signaling for help.

Narcotic painkillers have a euphoric effect that deadens team spirit and the ability to care about anything. They have a hypnotic effect that deadens alertness so that the user becomes too groggy for the challenges of sport or anything else. Addicts call it "nodding out."

OPIATES

As an athlete you need to know about the most dangerous painkillers. They are depressant drugs that slow many functions of the brain and central nervous system. The drugs are all related in structure to opium. They hook into the opiate receptors to cause the reward feelings you obtain from exercise.

The thalamic area of the brain has a high concentration of opiate receptors. Deep pain comes from the medial part of the thalamus. The amygdala area of the limbic system has the most opiate receptors. It causes the reward feelings: the "rush" or feeling of pleasure and warmth called euphoria.

Opiates have a sedative, depressant effect. Withdrawal from them is severe but not as bad as withdrawal from the late stages of alcohol addiction. You become addicted to opiates if you use them longer than needed in an emergency situation. Only a few weeks' use can be addictive.

Withdrawal from painkillers can be more painful than the pain you started treating. It can even cost your life. Breathing can be stopped by all depressant drugs; it is the extreme result of sedation.

MORPHINE

Some painkilling drugs are natural opioids. Morphine, made from the opium poppy, is used for terminally ill patients who suffer severe pain.

Morphine blocks the higher cortex, the thinking part of the brain. That interference leaves the emotional brain in control. Morphine binds with opiate receptors in parts of the central nervous system as a depressant. It masks pain and calms the emotional response to it. It can cause nightmares, euphoria, dizziness, and seizures. It is highly addictive. Taken with alcohol, it causes cross-addiction.

Morphine interferes with alertness, breathing, and heartbeat. It should not be used with head injuries. It can kill if taken with other depressants such as monoamine oxidase (MAO) inhibitors: cocaine, tricyclic antidepressants, alcohol, general anesthetics, sedatives, or hypnotics.

CODEINE

The opium poppy contains another painkilling drug, codeine. Used in cough and cold formulas as well as for pain, it is a dangerous depressant drug and is banned by the IOC.

HEROIN

Athletes who use narcotic painkillers are asking for big trouble. They risk making their injuries much worse by not accepting the message of pain. Users of heroin risk putting themselves in danger because of a damaged mental state.

Heroin is a semisynthetic opioid; it is morphine that has been chemically altered at the molecular level to make it stronger. It is much more addictive, and it is illegal, the only illegal narcotic in the United States. It is smuggled into the country. The word *heroin* comes from the German word for "hero"; it is so called because of the false sense of power it engenders. A false "hero" is deadened to personal risk. A true hero is brave in the face of danger; a false hero is stupid—meaning in a stupor or sleepy.

Dealers make extra money by cutting heroin with any white powder; often cornstarch, which is inexpensive, or quinine, which can have dangerous side effects. The mix is sold with as little as one percent real heroin for whatever the buyer is foolish enough to pay. After dilution with water, the heroin is cooked in a spoon. Then a needle and either a syringe or an eyedropper are used to inject it into a vein through a cotton filter.

Sometimes heroin addicts who have not paid their dealer are given a "hot shot," heroin that has been cut with a poison such as arsenic or strychnine, or even a cleansing agent.

Heroin users contract many infections: AIDS, hepatitis, abcesses, endocarditis, and septicemia are some of them.

The unsterile use of heroin is only one reason it is life-threatening. When a user overdoses, the medulla area of the brain suffers from central nervous system depression, which may be fatal. As a depressant, heroin is even more likely to cause death when used with other depressants such as alcohol or barbiturates. Heroin overdose also kills by causing collapse of the cardiovascular system.

Withdrawal from heroin causes addicts terrible pain. The electrical activity of the brain becomes oversensitive to pain signals. The chains of nerve cells that intensify pain cause them to experience "raw nerves."

METHADONE

Pharmaceutical companies have manufactured synthetic opiate narcotics. Methadone is a painkiller very close to morphine in molecular structure. It is used in treating heroin addicts to avoid painful withdrawal symptoms. They do not experience as much euphoria with methadone. It helps to keep them from committing crimes of violence in efforts to obtain heroin. However, addicts must eventually withdraw from the methadone.

Methadone has been used by athletes as a painkiller. It has not been established as a safe drug to use for maintenance of adolescent heroin addiction as it has for adults. It has a cumulative or additive effect that increases the depression. It is banned by the IOC.

OTHER NARCOTIC ANALGESICS

Narcotic analgesics can be used for acute pain that lasts days to weeks, but not for chronic pain. Opiate-based narcotics suppress the brain endorphins, which are the strongest painkillers of all—ten times stronger than morphine. The user feels more pain and uses more painkillers. The chronic pain actually gets worse, and the user becomes an addict.

Hydromorphone hydrochloride is a semisynthetic opioid that is sold as Dilaudid and under other brand names. It binds with opiate receptors in the brain, brainstem, and spinal cord to mask pain and to alter the emotional response to pain. It is a banned drug.

Dilaudid also slows breathing, which is very dangerous for athletes, and it causes the euphoric effect. It is mainly effective as a painkiller if taken before pain is intense. It causes urine buildup and constipation and strains the heart. It can also cause nausea, vomiting, and, in large doses, seizures.

Percodan is a combination of aspirin and oxycodone. An addictive semisynthetic opioid, it works like morphine.

Remember that opiate and opioid painkillers should not be taken with monoamine oxidase (MAO) inhibitor drugs such as cocaine. Some combinations of painkillers work against each other.

Meperidine (trade name, Demerol) is an IOC-banned drug. A synthetic opioid, it is used to relieve moderate to severe pain. It reacts badly with MAO drugs such as crack. It can cause feelings of unreality, with hallucinations, depression, slowed heartbeat, ringing in the ears, swollen face, skin rash, itchy skin, uncontrolled muscle movements, tremors, and confusion. If that is not enough to make you avoid it, it can also cause heart trouble, breathing depression, dizziness, sleepiness, muscle twitching, nausea, vomiting, and constipation.

Propoxyphene hydrochloride (trade name, Darvon) is another synthetic opioid. It binds with opiate receptors in many parts of the central nervous system. It is only about as effective as aspirin for pain relief. It is sometimes used by athletes to cut down the amount of steroids in their urine before a drug test.

With caffeine or amphetamines, Darvon can cause seizures. It decreases alertness but causes excitement and interferes with sleep. It is addictive and cross-addictive with other depressants: other opiate narcotics, alcohol, or barbiturates. Sometimes it is mixed with aspirin and acetaminophen to increase the painkilling effect.

BARBITURATES

Barbiturates ("barbs") come in colored capsules: red (Red Devils), blue (Blue Devils), yellow (yellow jackets or yellows), and blue and red. They are also called by brand names.

Athletes use barbiturates as muscle relaxants and anti-anxiety agents to avoid feeling stressed by competition. However, they hurt sports performance by interfering with motor cordination, and they have many dangerous side effects. Barbiturates are sedative-hypnotic drugs. As depressants, an overdose alone or combined with other depressants can be lethal.

Athletes on barbiturates experience delusions of greatly improved abilities. As a result many athletes overtrain or compete before they are ready. Many injuries result from taking risks because of delusions of enhanced performance.

Barbiturates are prescribed as anticonvulsants for victims of seizures because they raise the seizure threshold in the motor cortical area of the brain. They interfere with impulse transmission from the thalamus to the cortex. Used with MAO inhibitors such as crack, the depressant effect lasts longer. Use of *butabarbital sodium* is excessively dangerous.

Barbiturate poisoning can make the user turn blue from cyanosis and have clammy skin. The pupils of the eyes contract. Coma and respiratory depression can lead to death. Withdrawal symptoms can be very severe.

CHAPTER 6

Steroids and Other Hormones

The hormonal balance of the human body is very fragile and can be tipped easily. The result can be irreparable damage.

The hormonal changes caused by use of anabolic androgenous steroids have ruined the performance and potential of many athletes. Most took them for the *ergogenic* or performance-enhancing effect.

Anabolic androgenous steroids (AASs) have killed many athletes who had no idea what they were putting into their bodies. Now the facts are pretty common knowledge, but you need to understand how your body reacts to hormonal interference to understand the dangers and risks of use.

Your body makes and balances its own hormones. A hormone is a biochemical transmitter that is released by a cell. It travels along neurons to change another part of the body at its receptors. There are quite a few kinds of hormones. This chapter is about the hormones that affect growth.

Growth hormones affect every cell in your body. They affect muscle development, bone growth, and mental processes. Your teenage growth achieves a total makeover of your brain and body, transforming you from a child into an adult.

Growth hormone is secreted by the pituitary gland. In girls, the ovaries are changed so they can make the hormone *estrogen*. Estrogen helps develop breasts and allows an ovum to be released to the uterus each month. The lining of the uterus becomes soft to protect the ovum in case it is impregnated with sperm to create a pregnancy.

The ovum lives about forty-eight hours. During that time another female hormone, *progesterone*, adds nutrients to the lining of the uterus. If the girl does not become pregnant, the unused ovum and extra lining pass slowly out of her body. The few days during which that happens are called the *menstrual period*.

Girls start having menstrual periods at least one or two years after the breasts develop. At the first period, called menarche, the fast-growth period begins. The skeleton grows larger, then stronger.

Training hard lowers a girl's estrogen level, which can block menstruation for a while.

Boys' growth hormone is called *testosterone* because it comes from the testes and the pituitary gland. Girls produce testosterone in the ovaries and the pituitary gland, but less than boys.

Testosterone is the hormone that turns a boy into a grown man, with a lower voice and hair growth on his face and body.

Girls do not have enough testosterone to develop male characteristics unless they take anabolic androgenous steroids. If they do take AASs, they develop male hair growth patterns (hirsutism), lower voices, and enlarged clitoris. Menstruation can become irregular. They can lose interest in boys, get pimples on their bodies, and become very aggressive and even violent.

Drugs made of hormones or genetically engineered chemical structures copied from hormones are used by athletes for many reasons: to gain weight faster, to build muscles, or even to slow growth. What they get instead are health problems that do not go away when they stop taking the drugs.

This chapter will explain the side effects of AASs on normal growth processes, including muscle building.

Nutrients from foods become a balanced fuel for the human body. Steroid hormones and related hormone drugs used by athletes cause dangerous imbalances and only temporary advantages.

Stressing muscles but not overstressing them is what builds them. Three very different kinds of muscle contractions build muscle strength: *isometric*, *isotonic*, and *isokinetic*. With practice and good food you can build a strong and balanced muscle system.

Anabolic steroids are dangerous because they increase muscle strength quickly but tissues and tendons are not strengthened at the same rate. That creates a weakened, imbalanced body, putting the athlete at greater risk of injury. The National Football League has suffered many injuries because of steroid use. Both players who use and their opponents suffer because the users are more aggressive and even violent.

AAS use causes sexual aggressiveness that has led to criminal behavior like rape and murder. It has also resulted in the transmission of the AIDS virus. Just two weeks of steroid use allows testosterone levels to build up to risky levels.

Longer use of anabolic steroids snuffs out sexual interest.

Some users admit that their sexual drive has never returned even after withdrawal is many years behind them.

Some athletes have tried using various steroid drugs by mouth or injected into the bloodstream. They call it "stacking." It really is "stacking the cards against them." They do stacking for a few months, then go off steroids to try to avoid positive test results at competition time.

By 1988 an estimated 500,000 teenagers were injecting drugs such as steroids and heroin with needles and syringes potentially infected with the AIDS virus. They are being called the "lost generation."

Anabolic steroids cause heart attacks, myocardial infarction, and stroke, which can result in death. Sharing needles to inject steroids can also mean sharing death from AIDS.

Teenagers on steroids stop growing because the long bone growth plates are forced to close early. It is called premature epiphyseal closure. They develop severe acne, much worse than the usual teenage pimples caused by growth hormones. AAS users have it on the body as well as on the face.

Hair loss causes bald spots on athletes who use anabolic steroids. Steroids slow down fluid in the skin and shrink red blood cells. They inhibit the action of white blood cells that fight infections. The immune system is severely damaged. The skin can become thin and bruise easily.

GABA (gamma-aminobutyric acid) is a neurotransmitter with the special function of keeping nerves from becoming too stimulated. It binds with cell surface receptors for that purpose. Steroids have been found to bind with GABA receptors and change the shape. When the receptor shape is changed, the cell switches from hormone-sending to interference with the central nervous system, masking pain and anxiety.

AASs build muscles that contain extra salt and water. Athletes lose both strength and weight as the effects wear off. Does anyone really want saltwater muscles?

Digested protein foods become amino acids in peptide linkage. Amino acids are an important part of the hormones your body makes. Absorbed into the bloodstream right away, they work as biochemical structures that carry nutrients. They act as natural pain relievers, ten times stronger than morphine.

Amino acids work as neurotransmitters. They can also act as antibodies that fight disease. The dry weight of your body cells is three quarters amino acids.

Your body produces natural steroid hormones to handle stress and infection. Adding drugs with steroid hormone structures upsets the chemical balance. Imbalance eventually leads to poisoning and even death.

Drugs that have a molecular structure called the steroid nucleus are grouped as steroids. All hormones are steroids. They include the male hormone testosterone and the female hormones estrogen and progesterone.

The steroid molecular structure is used as the basis of many synthetic drugs. Steroids that affect the whole body, as AASs do, are called systemic steroids.

Steroids are among the strongest drugs available. They have many dangerous side effects. They should be used only for emergency treatment for very severe problems and only with medical monitoring for side effects.

The adrenal gland produces adrenaline, the hormone used to prepare the body for self-defense. The outer layer of the adrenal gland is called the cortex. The drug cortisone is named after the cortex, which produces it.

Some athletes have thought cortisone was an anabolic steroid, but it is not. Cortisone and certain other drugs are the opposite of anabolic: catabolic. Catabolic steroids do not build muscle, they reduce it. Cortisone and drugs with similar structures are used as antiinflamatory drugs. They are also used after surgery. If cortisone is used longer than needed for emergency use, it can cause muscles to be destroyed.

If catabolic steroids like cortisone or corticosteroids are used with anabolic androgenous steroids, they can cause kinetic muscle imbalance and rupture tendons under stress.

Steroids raise blood pressure and blood cholesterol to dangerous levels. If blood cholesterol rises above 200 mg/dl it slows blood flow to the brain and body and damages arteries, causing coronary heart disease.

Foods with empty calories, called "junk foods" because they lack essential nutrients, raise the blood cholesterol. Avoid junk foods to gain a competitive edge.

The most compact useful food for supplying balanced amino acids is the egg. The egg raises blood plasma levels of amino acids. That means more essential biochemical structures going to bat for you. The egg contains a balance of nutrients, especially lecithin, which prevents it from raising the blood cholesterol more than 2 percent. Two percents add up, however, so eat eggs within reason.

High-density lipoprotein (HDL) is another constituent of the blood. You need more of it because it helps to clean the arteries. Exercise and vitamins increase HDL cholesterol. Drugs, including growth hormone drugs and alcohol, waste HDL cholesterol so that the arteries can become more clogged.

To cope with drugs, the pressure to perform well in sports, and the stresses of training, and to grow and build your strength, you need extra *stress amino acids* from a well-balanced selection of foods.

Stress amino acids have a branching structure. They are called *branched chain amino acids*, or BCAAs. Besides fighting stress damage, BCAAs improve muscle metabolism, which builds stronger muscles. They also act as fuel for energy output.

The three BCAAs are *isoleucine, leucine,* and *valine.* They are most balanced when eaten in foods. Supplements are overprocessed versions. Isoleucine metabolizes fats and carbohydrates and helps absorb and store protein. Lack of isoleucine causes tremors and muscle twitches. Stress from a workout causes a lessening of isoleucine in your body. You need to eat BCAA-containing foods to replace what you have lost.

Leucine stimulates protein synthesis in the muscles. Leucine is necessary for anabolic reactions and for protein storage. When you are under stress, as when you train hard or take drugs, your body uses leucine in a special protective way. It is used to make *alanine*, an amino acid that helps metabolize glucose, the energy fuel used by your skeletal muscles and brain.

The BCAA *valine* metabolizes carbohydrates. Valine is a natural stimulant. Insufficient valine results in a negative hydrogen balance, which shows up as neurological problems. Valine improves muscle metabolism, tissue repair, and nitrogen balance.

Anabolic muscle cell receptors are made to receive natural testosterone. Testosterone increases the output of RNA, which permits better protein synthesis. The anabolic steroids also improve protein use and nitrogen storage, but with great risks.

BCAAs are found in foods that our bodies have evolved to handle with astounding efficiency. They accomplish the same growth and performance tasks without the dangerous side effects.

Exercise causes testosterone loss, but then stimulates its production. Steroids cut off the production of natural testosterone. Better testosterone production improves protein synthesis.

The hypothalamus region of the brain triggers the pituitary gland. The pituitary makes *gonadotropin*, which also enhances testosterone production. So you start with losses from exercise and increase your supply while you recover.

During drug-free exercise, muscle strength, tissue strength, and tendon strength are developed in balance, which helps to prevent ruptures and other severe injuries.

In boys, use of anabolic steroids interferes with the natural production of testosterone. The voice becomes high-pitched instead of deepening. The testes shrink. The drug can also cause abnormal sperm, which can result in infants with birth defects even twenty years later.

Boys can develop breasts, sometimes discharging a clear fluid. Many boys take anabolic steroids hoping to improve their looks. They are in for a shock.

At the 1988 Olympic Games in Seoul, South Korea, Ben Johnson, a Canadian sprinter, won a gold medal, running the 100-meter dash in 9.79 seconds. He was stripped of his medal and suspended because a urine test proved he had been using the steroid Stanazonol. The International Amateur Athletic Federation (IAAF) banned him from international competition for two years. Carl Lewis of the United States was awarded the 100-meter gold medal instead.

The world media handled the matter as a cheating scandal but did not warn of the dangers of steroid use.

Athletes kept looking for ways of cheating on the tests, not realizing they were only cheating themselves.

Johnson had to pass six tests for steroids during the two-year suspension. Chief Justice Charles Dubin was appointed to investigate steroid use among Canadian athletes. In June 1990 Dubin made public his 638-page report. He blamed not only the athletes but their trainers and coaches and sports governing bodies. He said that tougher controls and heavier penalties should be established.

Because Johnson had received such severe punishment while so many other athletes had gotten by with use of steroids, Dubin recommended that the bans against Johnson be lifted. The IAAF suspension and the Canadian Olympic Association (COA) lifetime ban were both lifted so that Johnson could compete again.

By January 1991 Johnson had lost his saltwater muscles and was completely off steroids. He finished second in his first official race since the Olympics, running the 50-yard dash in 5.77 seconds, just 0.16 second slower than the world record.

The Track Athletic Congress (TAC), which governs United States track and field events, started year-round drug testing, but athletes living over 75 miles from testing centers were exempted. Because of the exemption 395 athletes were not tested and only 246 were. In February 1991 the TAC hired a company to do the extra testing.

Meanwhile, the July, 1990, *Track and Field News* featured a two-page interview with TAC Executive Director Ollan Cassell. Like the media in the Johnson case, Cassell mentioned the use of drugs such as ephedrine and steroids in cheating for the advantage of enhancing performance. However, he showed no understanding of the need to protect athletes from the devastating side effects of those drugs. Cassell stated: ". . . I think that at the same time we want to have a program in drug testing that is respected by everyone, that is fair, and that provides assurance to the athletes that they're competing on natural ability. Not on drug ability, not on a doctor's ability." *T&FN* asked, "How do you feel about the public perception that TAC is ridiculously suspending athletes for taking cold medicines and vitamins?" Cassell responded: "Some of those things are unfortunate because the levels of some of the athletes have been very high in the ephedrine area. They've complained about it, but the scientific studies indicate that when you get beyond a certain level, there's an advantage that you gain."

Steve Courson had a nine-year National Football League (NFL) career with two Super Bowl titles. In 1988 he found out that he had developed a rare heart condition from taking anabolic androgenous steroids. The disease had enlarged his heart and weakened its walls. He was scheduled for a heart transplant.

While he was on the waiting list for the transplant Courson traveled around the United States to warn other athletes of the dangers of steroid use. An Associated Press release quoted him:

> Our generation of athletes never had the benefit of making an informed choice. Our measuring stick for what they do is based solely on their performance, therefore it lends to the predicament of taking a performance-enhancing drug.

Athletes now have information available. You can choose to protect your heart, mind, body, and sports career. It is your responsibility to learn about any drug you might be tempted to take. Weigh the risks seriously or you might pay with your life.

The Associated Press reported that despite Ben Johnson's suspension for steroid use, two track and field athletes had tested positive for steroids. Both held records and were risking their chances of competing in the 1991 World Championships in Tokyo and the 1992 Olympics at Barcelona, Spain. Butch Reynolds had tested positive for the steroid nandrolone and Randy Barnes for the steroid methyltestosterone. Reynolds has held the 400-meter record and Barnes the shot put record. They were each given two-year bans.

"Track nuts," as the really committed fans call themselves, were disappointed. Those two athletes seemed to have let them down. Later it was reported that the urine samples had not been sealed in the presence of the athletes, in violation of IAAF rules. They both had had good test results before as well as after the "positive" tests.

The method of testing may be changed from urine tests to hair analysis. Experts are working on ways to make it more reliable. The thing to keep in mind is that there is no way to get around the penalties for steroid use.

DIURETICS

Regardless of the risks, athletes often use diuretics before being tested to dilute the amount of AASs and other drugs in their urine samples. Diuretics are also used to increase weight loss, so the athlete can compete in a lighter weight class. They can cause serious side effects, so they are banned by the IOC.

Diuretics cause loss of electrolytes (sodium, potassium,

chloride). They cause dehydration, muscle cramps, and a drop in blood pressure. They interfere with brain processes.

Diuretics are of several structural types, based on which part of the brain they affect. The first type is the *carbonic anhydrase inhibitor*, which causes elimination of sodium, potassium, bicarbonate, and water. It interferes with blood and can cause anemia. It acts as a depressant, causing drowsiness and confusion. It lowers eye pressure, causing temporary nearsightedness. It causes nausea, vomiting, and weight loss, makes breathing difficult, and causes asthma attacks. It is banned by the IOC and other sport associations.

A *loop diuretic* slows the return of sodium and chloride at the loop of Henle in the kidney, causing dangerous loss of fluids and electrolytes. It can cause dizziness, headaches, temporary loss of hearing, and muscle weakness and cramps.

The third type of diuretic is called *potassium-sparing*. It acts on the *distal tubule* to slow the release of potassium and the return of sodium.

Potassium-sparing diuretics are sometimes used with potassium-wasting diuretics. They increase the buildup of potassium when potassium supplements or salt substitutes have been taken.

Thiazide diuretics slow sodium return, increasing the output of urine, sodium, and water. They can cause dehydration, fluid and electrolyte imbalances, sensitivity to light, skin rashes, and anemia. Some thiazide-like diuretics cause similar problems.

About ten combinations of diuretics are used. They mainly combine hydrochlorthiazide with spironolactone in various doses, causing double trouble.

HUMAN GROWTH HORMONE

Somatotropin is human growth hormone (hGH); HGH is a synthetic form. Both can cause allergic reaction, diabetes, and gigantism in high doses. HGH is used as an anabolic steroid substitute because it blends with natural growth hormone made in the pituitary area of the brain.

Until 1985 athletes used only hGH, which is obtained from dead brains. At that time, genetic engineers synthesized the natural hormone. Four boys had contracted a dead person's disease from hGH and died. It was taken off the legal market in the United States.

Many athletes still prefer hGH and import it from other countries. They will do anything to win, but they eventually lose from using hGH. It can cause AIDS or other diseases from the dead donor.

Damage can be done to the heart muscle by either form of human growth hormone from gaining weight too fast. The weight-bearing skeletal muscle system is also harmed. The drugs can cause joint-cartilage problems, diabetes, and arthritis.

The metabolic and systemic side effects of hGH and HGH include gigantism or acromegaly. The drug makes bones grow longer, which results in huge hands and feet and a long chin. The nose spreads, and the lips and fingers swell because of overgrowth of soft tissue.

HUMAN CHORIONIC GONADOTROPIN

Another peptide hormone is human chorionic gonadotropin (hCG). It stimulates the production of androgen in the testes. For testing purposes it is considered the same as taking anabolic steroids by mouth or injection. It is banned by the IOC and other sport associations. The drug can cause headache, depression, irritability, restlessness, and fatigue. It is especially dangerous to 10- to 13-year-olds. It causes water retention and female-like bodies as steroids do.

ERYTHROPOIETIN

Erythropoietin (EPO) is a glucoprotein hormone produced in human kidneys. It regulates erythrocyte synthesis. Athletes use EPO to increase red blood cells, which carry oxygen, hoping to improve endurance. Actually it wastes iron, causing deficiency. The red blood cells increase until the blood thickens, which can cause hypertension, clots and heart attacks, thrombosis, and stroke.

In the last two years, sixteen bicyclists from Holland have died at very young ages in otherwise very good condition. They all used EPO.

EPO is injected, so needle sharing can infect users with AIDS. EPO can also cause headaches and seizures because of its effects on the central nervous system, nausea, vomiting and diarrhea, and skin rashes.

CORTICOTROPIN

Corticotropin (ACTH) is a pituitary hormone used by athletes to increase corticosteroid levels in the blood. It takes the place of the natural hormone and stimulates the adrenal cortex to give up its storage of several hormones. For testing purposes it is considered the same as taking corticosteroids by mouth or injection. It is banned by the IOC.

ACTH can cause seizures, headaches, and dizziness; personality changes with mood swings, depression, and even psychosis; eye problems (cataracts or glaucoma);

ulcers, nausea, and vomiting. Girls' menstrual periods become irregular.

ACTH interferes with nitrogen balance and wastes calcium and potassium. It retards healing and causes acne and heavy sweating. It actually can cause loss of muscle mass and stunt growth.

VASOPRESSIN

Vasopressin (Pitressin) is another pituitary hormone used to stimulate growth hormones. It is also called antidiuretic hormone (ADH).

It can cause water intoxication, which can result in seizures, coma, and death. The early symptoms of water intoxication are sleepiness, headache, and confusion.

Some people have allergic reactions, asthma attacks, fever, rash, and swelling from water retention. In girls it can cause cramps in the uterus. Both boys and girls can have abdominal cramps, nausea, vomiting, and diarrhea. It can cause heart attack (angina) and hypertension.

CLONIDINE

Clonidine is used by athletes to stimulate growth hormones. It depresses the central nervous system and can interact with any other depressant to make the effects fatal. Clonidine also causes a hypertensive response and vivid dreams when used with beta blockers such as propranolol, or with tricyclic antidepressants or MAO inhibitors such as cocaine.

BETA BLOCKERS

Beta blockers are used by athletes to stimulate growth hormones. *Propranolol hydrochloride* (Inderal and others) is a beta-adrenergic blocker. It reduces the heart muscle's need for oxygen. It blocks the neurotransmitter catecholamine, which would otherwise create fast heartbeat and high blood pressure.

Propranolol is a depressant that can cause fatigue, vomiting, hallucinations, and vivid dreams. Propranolol with epinephrine can cause severe vasoconstriction. It can worsen medical problems such as allergies, asthma, diabetes, and heart trouble.

LEVODOPA

Levodopa (L-dopa) is used by athletes to stimulate growth hormone. It has a very strong effect on the central nervous system. It can cause both aggressive and suicidal behavior. L-dopa interferes with body movements and can cause tremors and twitching. L-dopa can cause nausea, vomiting, and loss of appetite leading to malnutrition problems.

L-dopa causes mood changes with nervousness, anxiety, euphoria, severe depression, and suicidal tendencies. It can drive an athlete out of touch with reality and into hallucinations and delirium. Memory fades, and mental problems develop.

L-dopa can cause diabetes and acromegaly. Liver and kidney function is diminished.

Bromocriptine mesylate (Parlodel) activates dopamine receptors and intensifies the effects of L-dopa. It causes a wide range of central nervous system problems: dizziness, confusion, hallucinations, uncontrollable body movements, delusions and manic behavior, insomnia, fatigue, depression, blurred vision, and abdominal problems.

ARGININE

Arginine is an essential amino acid taken by athletes who hope to increase growth hormone levels. Arginine acts as a vehicle for nitrogen, which improves muscle metabolism. The high-energy chemicals used by muscles are made from arginine; they are guanidophosphate, phosphoarginine, and creatine.

Arginine loading (use of supplements) is poorly absorbed in the blood, and growth hormone levels show little or no change. Argenine injections of 20–25 g release growth hormone. Argenine blocks pain relievers and antibacterials but seems to promote wound healing and nitrogen balance.

L-ornithine supplements taken by mouth can be made into arginine in the body. Some athletes take 3000 mg tablets morning and night as part of a growth hormone releasing supplement. It is not considered enough to stimulate growth. But too much ornithine causes depression, swollen legs (edema), and hypothyroidism.

The safest way to get enough arginine or any of the other amino acids is through a well-balanced diet. Foods rich in arginine are milk and cheese, eggs, nuts, and wheat germ.

CHAPTER ◇ 7

Antianxiety Drugs

Antianxiety agents and other psychoactive drugs damage neurochemical balance. They wear down receptors and nerves and strain the body. That makes it even more difficult to manage stress in any form. When you take drugs you are starting a jittery, nervous, stressful existence.

You can lower the noise on a stereo by turning a knob. Your body has a limbic system that functions like that knob. It keeps the sound waves of noise from bothering you. Noise is stress. Too much stress damages the limbic system. You can become easily irritated by noise and other stresses.

Once your mood has been disturbed by stress, it becomes even more sensitive. More physical damage occurs even if you stop using drugs because of the stress. To cope with drugs and sports, you need to learn to relax and handle stressful situations carefully.

Using antianxiety agents can make your brain and body less able to handle the chemicals produced by stress. If you depend on antianxiety agents to calm you, you will not be developing the coping techniques that you need. Find ways of coping that work for you, and make them into habits so that the rest of your life will be easier to manage. Chapter 11 will give you some ideas.

Drugs that depress or slow the central nervous system are called depressants, or sedative-hypnotics. Like all psychoactive drugs, they waste nutrients that are needed for sports performance.

Depressants in small doses can make you feel calmer. In larger doses they block critical thinking ability and can put you to sleep, even permanantly. You can die from any depressant drug because depressants slow the breathing centers in the brainstem.

Any depressant added to another makes the effect even worse. Many people have slowed themselves down to the point of death by taking alcohol with other depressants.

Athletes tend to push themselves to exhaustion during training and performance. Teenagers whose bodies are using enormous amounts of energy to grow can become very stressed. Anyone who is physically tired will react more strongly to alcohol and other depressants than when rested. Teenage athletes need to know the dangers of easily available depressant drugs. Alcohol causes more deaths of teenagers than any other drug.

If you become addicted to one depressant it can make you addicted to others. That is called cross-addiction. An addict must avoid all depressants.

Depressant drugs slow all the neurons in your brain and interfere with every cell in your body. They can be addictive, and withdrawal symptoms can lead to death.

Damage to the neurons of the brain causes mental problems. Depressants block memory, insight, and judgment. They interfere with reasoning. People on depressants become confused about their own identity and the identity of others. They lose track of where they are. They lose their sense of timing.

Some drugs make people more aggressive by inhibiting the part of the brain that controls violence. Many teenagers have been raped by dates made aggressive by drinking alcohol. Even more have been easily seduced because their protective shyness and common sense have been blocked. A few moments of careless behavior can transmit the AIDS virus, which kills.

ALCOHOL

Alcohol is the central nervous system depressant *ethanol*. It is the drug most abused by athletes. In 1990 research teams from the University of California at Los Angeles and the University of Texas announced a breakthrough. They had found a chemical receptor where alcohol activates reward-seeking behavior by blocking inhibitions. It is a receptor for the catecholamine neurotransmitter dopamine and is called D2.

The researchers found that almost 70 percent of alcoholics have an abnormal D2 receptor in the brain. As part of the chromosomal arrangements parents combine when they conceive a child, the D2 receptor gene becomes either a strength or a weakness with which their child must learn to cope. The gene is also found in 20 percent of persons who do not drink.

In the United States over 28 million people have alcoholic parents. If you have relatives who have developed alcohol addiction you are at high risk for developing it yourself if you drink. Of course, you can totally eliminate the risk by not drinking alcohol at all.

When alcohol fills the D2 receptors, fine movements are not possible. The D2 receptor slows fine movements.

Dopamine, including the subtype D2, is made from the amino acid *tyrosine.* We get tyrosine from eating protein foods. Tyrosine prevents depression. It helps athletes cope with physical stress, builds adrenaline supplies for emergency use, and helps build epinephrine and norepinephrine.

Tyrosine has an antidepressant effect, but too much dopamine can lead to aggressive behavior. Alcoholics can become violently aggressive.

Neurotransmitter systems in your brain need to be balanced. Your brain will balance them if you provide it with balanced meals. Tyrosine obtained as part of a daily balanced diet helps in two ways. It helps you cope with physical exhaustion, and it builds up adrenaline supplies for emergency use and sport competition.

Alcohol turns off your brain's review of what you learn during daily training. It slows down rapid eye movement (REM) sleep during which your dreams process what you have learned during the day. Studies in 1990 showed that teenagers need at least 9½ hours of sleep every night. Lack of rest causes stress.

Alcohol gets into the blood fast when taken on an empty stomach. Having food in the stomach dilutes the alcohol and slows the rate at which it enters the bloodstream. But drinking water to dilute it does not make the alcohol leave the body any faster. No way is known to speed up the liver's processing of alcohol to get it out of the body. Seventy-five percent of all deaths of alcoholics are caused by cirrhosis of the liver, which becomes thickened and hardened from having to eliminate so many poisonous chemicals. Cirrhosis is the seventh most common cause of death among Americans.

The neurons of the brain are depressed by alcohol. The result is a slowing of every aspect of sports performance.

Low doses affect fine movement, control, and the ability to discriminate. Moods fluctuate, and emotions go wild. Higher concentrations of blood alcohol slow the cortex area of the brain, which destroys the euphoric effect.

Synaptic transmission is slowed, which slows your breathing. Alcohol in high concentrations can make you stop breathing and die.

Alcohol makes users easily provoked to anger, even hostile. Memory, concentration, critical thinking, and judgment are slowed. Study becomes difficult. Stress increases at every level of damage, making the next drink more harmful.

The worst effect of alcohol on an athlete may be interference with the sense of balance. An athlete who has had alcohol may feel calmer but be less steady.

Alcohol slows reaction time, which must be immediate in most sports for effective play. Delayed responses can be dangerous.

An athlete needs quick and efficient motor nerves to send information to muscles. Alcohol slows your reflexes so you do not move with the trained responses you have worked hard to gain.

An athlete's ability to keep eyes on the ball or on other players, an ability known as visual tracking, can also be slowed for at least fourteen hours after heavy drinking.

You need nutrients to perform well in sports, but drugs waste many of them. Alcohol causes loss of thiamine and niacine, which can lead to serious problems in both the central and peripheral nervous systems.

Alcohol inactivates nutrients. It can diminish appetite so that you do not add enough essential nutrients. You can develop a protein deficiency. If your appetite is good, alcohol adds calories that turn into fat.

Alcohol wastes vitamin B_6 and folic acid, lack of which

can cause anemia. Alcohol washes out zinc, magnesium, and even some calcium in urination. It causes frequent urination.

Alcohol poisons the stomach, intestines, pancreas, liver, bone marrow, and heart. It breaks down into a toxic chemical called acetaldehyde. In some people the liver can further convert the acetaldehyde to vinegar and make it harmless. But if it does not break down, acetaldehyde causes brain damage, weakens the immune system, contributes to addiction, and wears out the liver.

Acetaldehyde reacts with brain neurotransmitters to form chemical structures call isoquinolines, which are very like the opiates and probably fit into the opiate receptors of the brain. As acetaldehyde damages brain and body, the isoquinolines can hook the drinker into masking the pain with more alcohol. That process makes the condition grow worse and worse.

Acetaldehyde causes damage to the DNA molecule, which is the source of inherited functions. It damages chemical bonds in protein and other large molecules. If oxidized, acetaldehyde can split into chemical fragments that can puncture cells, cause cancer, and wear out the system.

Withdrawal from alcohol can cause sleeping problems and nightmares. Even a strong athlete becomes weak and experiences muscle cramps and spasms. Withdrawal can cause vomiting, diarrhea, and appetite loss. It can increase the heartbeat to more than 100 per minute. It involves brain and body in a fight against the drug, with fever and heavy perspiration.

Those are only the early withdrawal symptoms. An alcoholic suffers even more.

Alcoholics suffering from withdrawal hallucinate; they see, hear, and feel things that are not there. They become paranoid, thinking people are out to get them. All their senses are depressed, causing delirium—uncontrollable seizures of spasms, fits, and convulsions about 48 hours after the last drink.

TRANQUILIZERS

The majority of antianxiety prescriptions in the United States are for benzodiazepines, or tranquilizers. Valium is the most widely used of all the benzodiazepines. Women are more sensitive to both alcohol and benzodiazepines because they have a different enzyme level than men that makes it harder to handle even low doses.

Benzodiazepines have been prescribed for athletes to relax muscles and improve lower back pain as well as to relieve anxiety. They cure nothing; they only mask muscle pain and emotional problems that should be solved.

Learning to relax and tackle problems a little at a time helps most sports anxiety. Developing a more positive way of thinking helps the most. For instance, concentrating on doing your personal best rather than on beating the competition is less stressful. Your coach or P.E. teacher should be able to advise you about developing useful attitudes.

Benzodiazepines interfere with the thalamus, hypothalamus, and limbic system of the brain. They are depressants and have many dangerous effects on both brain and body. Athletes use benzodiazepines to calm down and cope with stress. They make the athlete think performance has been great when it was only ordinary. Sports skills are slowed. Mental abilities are confused. Muscles are weakened. Sleep loss makes anxiety worse. Headaches and nausea are common effects. Menstruation is interfered with in girls. Sexual function is diminished in boys.

An overdose of benzodiazepine causes low blood pressure and heart and breathing depression. The result can be coma and death.

The worries, sleeplessness, and muscle spasms caused by addiction to and withdrawal from benzodiazepines indicate that the potential harm outweighs the potential benefits.

The most widely used tranquilizer, Valium (diazepam), is a long-acting benzodiazepine. It is a depressant and therefore very dangerous when taken with other depressant drugs. Many people have died from combining alcohol and Valium.

Valium is sometimes prescribed for athletes to relieve skeletal muscle spasm. Valium can make it hard to breathe. It can cause fatigue and weakness, confusion, skin rash, and itchiness. It is definitely not a help to athletic performance. It can lead to coordination problems, dizziness, and coma. It is banned by the IOC.

Withdrawal from benzodiazepines can involve psychotic behavior, hallucinations, muscle cramps, inability to sleep, and violent behavior. Withdrawal symptoms may not occur for up to twelve days after stopping use, and they can last for weeks.

The short-acting benzodiazepines such as Xanax leave the body more quickly, but they are more addictive than the longer-acting ones.

BETA BLOCKERS

Beta blockers are used as antianxiety drugs and to reduce tremors before competition. They are sometimes prescribed for athletes who are trembling or "choking" because of emotional tension. They are also prescribed to help athletes relax, sleep, and reduce muscle spasms.

Beta blockers waste the athlete's energy resources. They block the breakdown of carbohydrates and fats. They can cause heart attacks, strange and frightening nightmares, and hallucinations. The beta blockers are banned by the IOC.

Beta blockers work mostly on beta 1 receptors, which are in the kidneys and heart. Beta 2 receptors, in the arteries, lungs, and liver, are blocked if an increased dose or overdose is taken.

Beta blockers stimulate beta adrenergic receptors. They cause fast heartbeat and breakdown of fats and carbohydrates, which leaves less energy for sports. They can cause hair loss and stomach upset. Boys lose their sexual drive.

If an athlete has asthma, a beta blocker can cause bronchospasms or difficult breathing. Blood pressure can be lowered and heart rate slowed. Heart failure can be caused by beta blockers.

CHAPTER 8

Psychomotor

Stimulants

Athletes use cocaine as a psychomotor stimulant thinking it will improve their performance as an ergogenic aid. But in eighteen months of cocaine use, more teenagers have brain seizures, become violent to others, or kill themselves than do adults who have used cocaine for seven years.

Even small amounts of cocaine interfere with many vital brain and body systems. Two lines of cocaine can kill you. About 1,700 deaths from cocaine were reported in 1987 alone.

Cocaine prepares the body to deal with emergencies. It is a sympathominetic drug; that is, it mimics stimulation of the sympathetic nervous system. Cocaine blocks norepinephrine transmitters when they are returning to their receptors. They are abandoned in the synaptic cleft between nerve endings, where they break down into new chemical structures. One type of structure is adrenochrone, which can form adrenolutin. Adrenolutin causes hallucinations and tricks the senses.

Cocaine is a monoamine oxydase inhibitor (MAO or MAOI). Many prescription and OTC drugs have label warnings against their use with MAO inhibitors.

Cocaine stimulates the emotional center of the brain, the nucleus accumbens, which is what causes the strong craving for the drug.

Cocaine causes dopamine to stay in the synaptic cleft, which makes the limbic system overactive. The result can be confusion, agitation, hallucinations, and euphoria.

Cocaine slows down returning serotonin, the body's calming neurotransmitter. When it is blocked it causes severe headaches, worry, and restlessness.

Cocaine makes the heart beat faster, which increases the need for oxygen. Athletes experience oxygen debt. If you are without oxygen you faint in seconds.

Cocaine also wastes blood glucose, which is a form of sugar made in the body from carbohydrates. An athlete burns glucose as fuel for energy. Glucose is the main source of energy for the brain too. Fainting can be caused by glucose shortage.

Your brain is always active. Unless it has stored enough glucose, glycogen, and the high-energy adenosine triphosphate (ATP) as well as oxygen, it will be permanently damaged.

Coma and death occur if the brain is without oxygen or glucose for several minutes, as when someone drowns or chokes, or uses cocaine.

Cocaine releases catecholamines, which invade the sympathetic nervous system and overstimulate the receptor neurons. Chest pain, syncope, seizures, and tachycardia can result.

Cocaine causes hypertension, which can lead to death from stroke if arteries to the brain close.

Cocaine deaths have resulted from delirium, a frightening combination of delusions, illusions, and hallucinations. Less severe anxiety and agitation can also be caused by cocaine.

Cocaine schizophrenic psychosis is the term for another form of cocaine-caused death. The user becomes feverish, strong, and even murderous after only a small amount of cocaine. He may die from intense nerve stimulation that causes heart failure.

Cocaine withdrawal causes muscles to twitch, ache, and become exhausted from glucose and oxygen deprivation. The body is racked with chills. The mind becomes depressed and full of delusions, hallucinations, and suicidal thoughts.

Years after withdrawal, former addicts can experience cocaine-induced panic attacks. A panic attack can include fast heartbeat, heavy sweating, hyperventilating, and tremors. Brain waves are patterned very much like those of an epileptic seizure. Panic attacks have also happened to users who stopped combining amphetamines with cocaine.

Cocaine dries the mucus in the bony sinuses behind the nose and constricts blood vessels. The bone is dissolved, the sinuses are inflamed, and the cartilage between the nostrils (the septum) is destroyed. As a result, the optic nerves that normally function in the sinus areas are destroyed too. That can lead to blindness.

CUTTING COCAINE

Cocaine is usually diluted with other substances, which is called *cutting*. Dealers make more money by adding white powders and crystals to the cocaine. They may use mannite, inositol, lactose, amino acids, cornstarch, sugars, caffeine, flour, boric acid, aspirin, or epsom salts as inert cuts (having no psychoactive drug effects).

Some inert cuts are dangerous. For instance, talc contains asbestos, a cancer-causing substance. If the talc is injected, it can cause blood clots.

Another dangerous inert cut is quinine, which is poisonous. It causes dizziness, visual and hearing problems, headaches, ringing in the ears, nausea, and diarrhea.

The inert list is pretty long, but there are far more dangerous cuts. Active cuts of cocaine include an amphetamine-like stimulant called Methedrine, which can be addictive and causes paranoia. Pemoline is used to make the cocaine high seem to last longer. It is almost the same type of stimulant as cocaine itself.

The most dangerous active cut is phencyclidine (PCP) or angel dust, which numbs the user to the pain of life-threatening injuries and can make the user murderous.

Cocaine itself has an anesthetic effect because it interferes with nerve transmission. To increase the pain-relieving effect, it is often cut with other anesthetics. Masking pain is especially dangerous for athletes. The anesthetic cuts include procaine, tetracaine, benzocaine, butacaine, and lidocaine. Each has its own side effects.

It could be fatal to combine a cocaine cut with an anesthetic drug, with alcohol, or another depressant. Drinking alcohol and using cocaine has caused many deaths. Alcohol combines with cocaine in the liver to form a new chemical called cocaethylene. It returns to the brain and binds with transmitters in the dopamine system, which increases the cocaine effects.

In 1986, Len Bias had just signed a million-dollar contract for five years to play professional basketball with the Boston Celtics. He was twenty-two years old. He celebrated with friends and died. According to *The Len Bias Story* by Lewis Cole, they had a six-pack of beer, some cognac, and an ounce of 88 percent pure cocaine. One of the party was asked if Len had had any alcohol, and he said "No, just a couple of beers." Beer is alcohol, and two beers is more alcohol. With cocaine that can be a deadly combination.

At first no one knew that Len used cocaine. When his body was examined, cocaine was found in his stomach. His heart appeared normal until a microscopic examination showed destruction of heart muscle fibers (myocardial fiber necrosis), proof that he had been a cocaine user for some time.

CRACK

Crack cocaine causes depression after the euphoria. The user feels an intense need to get the pleasure effect again. Moods go up and down like a yo-yo. The process is called "chasing the high." Users often start with "free stuff" given by dealers to get them hooked. The user then buys five-dollar "nickels," then forty-dollar "doves." Eventually the user needs two hundred dollars a day to get the same effect.

The Centers for Disease Control reported a 43 percent increase in teenagers infected by the AIDS virus between 1988 and 1989. It was believed that crack addiction leading to trade-offs of sex for drugs was the direct cause of the increase.

When the blood supply of glucose and oxygen is cut off from the brain it can cause a stroke. If it lasts a few minutes it leads to paralysis, coma, and even to death. Crack use has caused an increase in strokes among teenagers. Stroke can happen long after giving up the addiction. Cocaine interferes with the immune system and causes inflammatory processes. Other forms of cocaine are processed by the liver before getting to the brain. Crack goes to the brain in ten seconds.

The National Institute on Drug Abuse (NIDA) has studied the effect of crack on addicts. It was found to be more addictive than alcohol but less addictive than the nicotine found in tobacco.

The Addiction Research Center of Baltimore reports that one out of ten people who use alcohol becomes addicted. One out of six who use crack becomes addicted. Nine out of ten who use tobacco cigarettes become addicted.

AMPHETAMINES

Because of poorly designed studies that were made public in the early 1960s, athletes believed that amphetamines could improve performance. Recent, more accurate studies show that amphetamines mask fatigue rather than preventing it. They have also proved that amphetamines interfere with the cardiovascular (heart and blood) system. Release of norepinephrine can overstimulate the heart, causing death. Death from cerebral vascular hemorrhage (stroke) and hyperthermia (abnormally high fever) can also occur because of amphetamine use.

We have seen that psychomotor stimulants are released by the body when it is stressed. It is the "fight or flight" response that our ancestors developed as they survived dangers. All body systems are put on alert, and stored adrenaline is activated to stimulate the body.

Chemical engineers designed the molecular structure of amphetamines to be like adrenaline. Amphetamines stress the body to activate the sympathomimetic system, the self-defense system. But amphetamines can leave addicts feeling like cowards facing danger. Their muscles become tense, their hearts race, their hands sweat, they can even regress to childish activities and repeat movements again and again.

Amphetamine addicts lose their sense of purpose. They have great energy, but it is not directed. Sometimes they repeat a simple task over and over for days; the repetition is called *stereotypy*.

Amphetamine addicts can lose interest in their family, their friends, and even their sports. To be isolated without purposeful behavior puts the user at risk. To become too isolated can mean losing or never developing the social skills necessary to manage the stresses of life.

Amphetamines can be injected. Many infectious diseases including AIDS are passed by contaminated injection equipment.

Amphetamines mixed with MAO inhibitor drugs such as cocaine can cause hypertensive crisis (very high blood pressure).

Dexedrine (dextroamphetamine sulfate USP) or "dexies" have a label warning against use with MAOI drugs. If used with a tricyclic antidepressant it could overstimulate the brain. Darvon taken with dexies can cause convulsions and death.

Other dexies are Ferndex, Robese, and Spancap #1. They work mainly in the cerebral cortex and the reticular activating system. They waste the supply of norepinephrine stored in nerve terminals. They activate transmission of nerve impulses, giving a sense of excitement and alertness that classifies them as cerebral stimulants.

Dexies interfere with the central nervous system, causing restlessness, tremors, hyperactivity, talkativeness, insomnia, irritability, overstimulation, headaches, dizziness, and chills. They can cause sexual impotence. They interfere with psychomotor coordination to hurt sport performance.

Biphetamine and *diphetamine* ("Black Beauties") are prescription drugs containing half amphetamine and half dextroamphetamine. Combining those sympathomimetic drugs increases the effects of each and puts athletes at greater risk. Users become irritable, paranoid, and lose judgment and reasoning ability. They become hyperactive and can experience irregular pulse and very high blood pressure.

Black Beauty "look-alikes" are put together by "garage chemists" under uncontrolled and often unsterile conditions. Advertised in school newspapers and handed out free at schools, they have poisoned and killed their users.

Amphetamine-like substances that are also sympathomimetic drugs are sold as remedies for congestion, asthma, and overweight.

We discussed the dangers of ephedrine use in Chapter 4. A related substance, *phenylpropanolamine* (PPA) is also found in many OTC products, even some intended for children. Try to stay away from OTCs, and read the label carefully if you do use one.

CHAPTER 9

Athletes and
Smoking

Tobacco pollution, even from someone else's cigarette, can hurt your sports performance.

Perhaps an athlete hopes to sneak in a few drags behind the gym, in the fresh air, without hurting the day's sports performance. *Wrong.* Just one cigarette makes the heart race. Just one interferes with the flow of blood to the neuromuscular system and the flow of air to the lungs.

Those few drags weigh down the cilia (tiny hairs) so that they cannot clean the lungs of germs, chemicals, and mucus. Smokers get sick much more often than non-smokers because the cilia cannot filter out germs as easily.

Just one cigarette and the blood pressure rises; fingers and toes get cold. About 90 percent of the 4,000 chemicals in the tobacco stays in the lungs. That makes the brain, heart, air passages, and mouth tissues work harder to get back to clean living.

Cadmium from cigarettes can cause emphysema, a lung disease. Emphysema sufferers have to gasp for each breath. Nothing can be done to restore the injured tissues. Shortage of oxygen makes the heart work extra hard;

eventually it dies of exhaustion. Cadmium also affects the central nervous system, causing stress damage and hypertension.

Sometimes young cells keep dividing and destroy normal cells. A mass of such cells is called a tumor. The disease is called lung cancer, and it can be caused by smoking. The abnormal cell growth eventually blocks the bronchi, then destroys lung tissue. Cancerous cells may be carried by the lymph system to other organs, where they grow into new tumors.

Smokers have more gum disease than nonsmokers. Tobacco irritates the gum tissues. Smokers, especially women, lose more teeth and tooth-supporting bone than nonsmokers. Nicotine interferes with the gum cells' ability to attach to the roots of teeth.

Claudication (leg weakness) because of hardening of the arteries is common in smokers. Some 20,000 legs are amputated in the United States every year to save the lives of people with intermittent claudication.

Tobacco smokers require stronger painkillers than nonsmokers. Smoking interferes with antidepressant drugs. A doctor who asks what drugs you use needs to know about your smoking habits to prescribe effectively.

Smokers metabolize (use) caffeine faster than nonsmokers. Doctors at San Francisco General Hospital measured blood caffeine levels of smokers before and after withdrawal. After the subjects stopped smoking, the same amount of coffee caused much higher levels of blood caffeine, making persons trying to kick the habit very nervous. Smokers need to cut down on caffeine and tobacco at the same time.

Smoking wastes endorphins, the body's natural defenses against pain and anxiety. A smoker withdrawing from tobacco is more susceptible to pain and more apt to be worried and nervous until the supply of endorphins is restored.

NICOTINE

Nicotine is the most addictive drug not only in tobacco, but of all the drugs discussed in this book. It is a psychoactive drug. It is first a stimulant of the central nervous system and then a depressant. It changes important biochemicals in dangerous ways. It interferes with brain and muscle cells. Nicotine narrows the blood vessels; blood with nutrients including glucose and oxygen has trouble getting through. The heart must pump hard to force the blood to keep flowing.

Because tobacco does not cause drunken behavior the way alcohol does, most people do not realize how much damage the nicotine does. It goes immediately to the brain, causing euphoria. It has a calming effect and stimulates concentration for simple tasks. But nicotine blocks both short- and long-term memory. If your sport requires complicated thinking you will not do very well if you smoke.

Nicotine interferes with hormone production, which is especially dangerous for teenage development. It masks pain during use, but during withdrawal sensitivity to pain is increased. Nicotine puts you in a good mood, so you think you can ignore problems and they do not get solved. It makes muscles tense. Like cadmium, nicotine affects skin temperature, blood pressure, and heart rate.

Nicotine also binds with the dopamine receptors in the brain as do the opiates, cocaine, amphetamines, and alcohol. Dopamine receptors are the "reward system" that makes people addicted. Remember, nicotine is the most addictive of all the drugs.

EFFECTS ON HEALTH AND LIFE-STYLE

Anyone who has ever smoked has trouble smelling good foods, flowers, fresh air, and even the company of others. The smell of sweat can be calming, according to 1990 studies. If that does not inspire you, think about the dangers your nose can warn you about: smoke, leaking gas, spoiled food, dangerous air pollution, and even steroid users. The garlicky odor of a steroid user might tip you off to stay out of the way of a "roid rage."

Cigarette smoking makes it harder to think and harder to be physically active because of reduced breathing capacity. It depresses the sex drive and sex appeal. Cigarette smoking makes a person smell like an overfull ashtray and lose the special scent that attracts the opposite sex. It also interferes with good looks, which depend upon good circulation.

In a study of tobacco smokers by researchers of the National Cancer Institute, eating habits were found to be very poor. Cigarette smokers usually do not eat enough of the foods that make up a well-balanced diet. The more they smoke, the less they tend to eat nutritious foods. Because of poor diet, smokers risk many cancers that are not directly caused by tobacco.

Also, smokers use alcohol more than nonsmokers, so like alcoholics—or even as alcoholics—they fill up on empty calories.

Calories are burned faster during smoking, which makes some athletes think smoking will keep them lean. People who quit do gain five to ten pounds of body weight, but smoking tobacco causes fat to gather in the abdomen.

In 1989 the National Academy of Sciences raised the recommended daily allowance (RDA) of vitamin C for smokers from 60 mg to 100 mg. In 1990 it was discovered that smokers have 30 percent less vitamin E in their lung fluid than nonsmokers.

PASSIVE SMOKING

Tobacco contains 4,000 chemicals, which are released from the burning end of a cigarette and pollute the air as *sidestream smoke.* People who are captives of other people's smoking are called *passive smokers;* they have no control over the dangerous chemicals they breathe in.

One of those harmful chemicals is *cadmium,* which is stronger in the air than in the smoke that the smoker inhales. Breathing too much cadmium-polluted air causes bronchitis. The bronchial lining is irritated by the smoke. Hairlike structures called cilia usually trap carbon dioxide and other chemicals. Smoke particles wear the cilia out. The brain tries to make up for the loss by creating extra mucus to trap the pollution. The mucus needs to be coughed out, and the constant coughing leads to aching chest muscles and sore ribs.

Even passive smoking puts you at risk of developing lung cancer. Living with someone who smokes over a pack a day at home can double your risk.

The nicotine in tobacco, which breaks down into cotinine, is found in the blood of passive smokers. Another chemical in tobacco smoke, the deadly poison cyanide, breaks down into thiocyanate, which is also found in the blood of children who breathe in tobacco smoke. Children whose homes are polluted with tobacco smoke are twice as likely to contract pneumonia as those whose homes have clean air. Children, teenagers, and adults can die from pneumonia.

A room filled with cigarette smoke doubles the amount of carbon monoxide in the blood. It even poisons nonsmokers. It remains in the body as long as four hours after the person leaves the smoke-filled room. A lighted cigarette lying in an ashtray gives off more tar and nicotine particles than when it is being smoked.

The 15 percent of Americans who are allergic to tobacco smoke suffer when they breathe it. They can get eye irritations, congestion of the breathing passages, and asthma attacks that may happen more than an hour after breathing the smoke.

Benzene is another dangerous chemical in tobacco smoke. *Breakthrough* magazine in 1991 published an article adapted by Stephen Lyons from a report in the Boston *Globe*. The report warned that concentrations of benzene are much higher in smokers' homes than they are outdoors in polluted cities. Benzene is a by-product of the gasoline manufacturing and oil refining processes. It is used in many common materials: waxes, dyes, nylon, varnish, polystyrene, and linoleum.

Benzene forms while a cigarette burns. Smoking a pack and a half a day means inhaling ten times more benzene than nonsmokers normally breathe in.

Benzene levels are 50 percent higher in a smoker's house than in a nonsmoker's. Children who grow up with a smoking parent are twice as likely to develop leukemia. In 1987, when researchers discovered that benzene contributes to leukemia, factories were required to set the safety standard for benzene 90 percent lower, but even low levels of benzene exposure cause cancer.

SMOKELESS TOBACCO

Smokeless tobacco, called snuff or chewing tobacco, causes cancer of the mouth, throat, cheeks, and gums. It makes saliva fill the mouth of the user, which must be spit out constantly. Only a few weeks of *dipping* can cause white patches on the gums that can be cancerous. When a user smiles you can see wrinkled gums, discolored teeth with exposed roots, and bleeding, cracked lips.

The American Cancer Society published a public service brochure showing a boy with his face puffed out with mouth cancer. He has a tube in his nose, medals on his hospital gown, and a trophy in front of him. Below the picture is his short, sad story:

> A budding track athlete and a popular student, Sean Marsee started dipping when he was thirteen because he thought it was safer than smoking. After five years of dipping a can or more a day, he got mouth cancer. He had part of his tongue removed. At age nineteen he died, after writing a simple message on a pad of paper: "Don't dip snuff."

In Health magazine in 1990 stated that 39 percent of professional baseball players chew tobacco, and 46 percent of tobacco-chewing players have potentially cancerous mouth lesions.

MARIJUANA

Like tobacco smoking, each "hit" off a marijuana joint draws many harmful chemicals into the lungs. Marijuana has a higher concentration of cancer-causing chemicals than tobacco, including several psychoactive drugs.

Cannabis sativa (marijuana) contains more than 425 chemicals. Marijuana has more benzene in one hit of smoke than is in one "drag" of a tobacco cigarette. It also contains more ammonia, more hydrocyanic acid (HCN), and more acetaldehyde than tobacco. Marijuana contains at least 11 steroids, 50 hydrocarbons, 18 amino acids, 62 cannabinoids, 20 nitrogenous compounds, 12 fatty acids, 20 noncannabinoid phenols, 7 simple alcohols, and 20 simple acids.

Chapter 10 on pollutants and inhalants will further your understanding of the cancerous and otherwise harmful ingredients in marijuana. No athlete should even be around the sidestream smoke from marijuana joints.

Marijuana is dangerous in many ways. It can make sports unsafe for athletes for more than two weeks after use. It harms many sport skills. Depth perception is thrown off. The sense of timing is slowed. Muscle spasms interfere with performance. Memory is inhibited.

Other mental problems make marijuana users lose their will to try, to train, to finish. They become apathetic, easily frustrated, and more likely to quit.

Paranoia and hallucinations can occur. Aerobic lung capacity is weakened and reduced.

Some personality changes can remain after use. Severe depression, anxiety, and irritability are marks of marijuana withdrawal. They may remain as personality hang-ups. Withdrawal can also bring nausea, loss of appetite, and insomnia.

The strongest marijuana in the world is grown in the United States. Ninety percent of its marijuana is grown in five states: Missouri, Kentucky, Tennessee, California, and Hawaii. But the New England states grow hundreds of millions of dollars worth of marijuana too.

Drug dealers use cloning techniques to grow *sinsemilla*, a seedless marijuana that contains high levels of the psychoactive drug tetrahydrocannabinol (THC).

Ordinary marijuana has only one to two percent THC. Sinsemilla has been found to contain as much as 18 percent.

Researchers at the University of California at Los Angeles report that daily hits from one to three marijuana joints cause lung damage equal to five to fifteen tobacco cigarettes. A marijuana hit is breathed into the lungs and held there longer than a drag from a cigarette to increase the effect of the THC and other psychoactive ingredients.

The National Institute of Mental Health in 1990 reported identifying a receptor for THC in a protein on the surface of brain cells.

One area of the brain that marijuana interferes with is the hippocampus, the main part of the limbic system. The limbic system is responsible for information-processing through sensory experiences. It links them with the motivation to perform well. It also processes other types of learning and memory.

THC damages and destroys neurons and nerve fibers in the brain. It causes the same loss of cells seen in many old people. Marijuana smoking over several years can cause long-lasting memory problems. It blocks self-awareness, so users put up with problems they should be learning to solve.

Marijuana can suppress the part of the immune system that protects against herpes infections.

Sometimes *hashish* (marijuana resin) oil is added to marijuana, bringing the THC content to 34 percent.

Inhalants and the

Immune System

The drugs called inhalants are gases. Inhaled gases are very dangerous to the immune system. They also enter the bloodstream very quickly and damage the central nervous system and the neuromuscular system.

The air in people's homes can be seriously polluted with gases, especially when it is not exchanged. Even polluted outdoor air tends to have lower levels of pollutants than are found in most American homes.

One reason, besides the lack of fresh air, is that people are careless about following directions for storing gases. U.S. laws require manufacturers to place warnings on potentially harmful gases. It is your responsibility to follow their advice. If you do not, you may be harmed by invisible and often odorless vapors.

Inhaling gases reduces the oxygen needed by athletes to recover from oxygen debt. Inhalants can cause sneezing, coughing, nosebleed, fatigue, nausea, lack of coordination, and loss of appetite. Inhaled in concentrated amounts, they can cause violence and death.

The water we drink can contain toxic chemicals. Our bodies have to process toxic waste given off by bacteria. The food we eat can contain additives and traces of toxic herbicides and pesticides that are harmful to our biochemistry as well as that of plants and pests.

Because of environmental pollution we are at greater risk for dangerous effects from drugs. Remember that some chemicals, when mixed with others, become entirely different structures. Mixed drugs can also cause stronger and more dangerous reactions.

Athletic performance depends upon how well your body can get rid of toxins. The process of eliminating harmful substances including psychoactive drugs is called detoxification.

Your liver does most of the detoxification. It can be overworked and damaged by psychoactive drugs, including inhalants and other pollutants.

Heavy metals such as lead, mercury, cadmium, arsenic, aluminum, and nickel pile up in the brain and kidneys. You need a balanced diet with plenty of fiber to bind to those toxins so they are eliminated with the fibers.

Your kidneys need lots of water to eliminate ammonia, urea, and other toxins that result from protein breakdown. Your lymph system also helps your body get rid of the toxins it absorbs. High-fiber foods help bind bacteria and yeast toxins so they can be eliminated.

Some 100,000 chemicals in the environment can interfere with your health; more than 20 can harm your immune system.

Many of the chemicals are produced by factories. Some are from synthetic fabrics.

Sulfur dioxide and nitrogen dioxide (NO_2) are released into the air by power plants. NO_2 is the main pollutant in smog. It mixes with water in your body and breaks down into toxins that interfere with the disease-fighting macrophages of your immune system.

Lead and pesticides from air pollution have caused mental retardation. Pollutants such as tobacco and marijuana smoke can cause cancers.

Cigarette smoke has far higher levels of nitrites than are found in foods, according to a 1981 report by the National Academy of Sciences. Workers in the rubber, leather, and rocket fuel industries are exposed to high concentrations of nitrite pollution.

Burning of fossil fuels causes the release of natural or industrial sulfur and nitrogen oxides, which start the reactions that cause acid rain. Acid rain has destroyed forests, lakes and streams, and many forms of water life in many regions of the United States and Europe.

Exhausts from motor vehicles cause about 40 percent of the nitrogen oxide pollution. Utility fuel burning accounts for another 35 percent; industrial fuel burning, 12 percent, and other industrial processes less than 5 percent.

Acidic water dissolves copper and lead from pipes in water supply systems that can make it harmful to drink.

SNIFFING INHALANTS

Like other central nervous system depressants, including alcohol, inhalants can make users easy to seduce and abuse or rape. Under the influence of inhalants, users may do things they would never do with the good-judgment part of their brain functioning.

During 1990 more teenagers than ever before started using inhalants. The risks from use are higher than ever because of the dangerous levels of gases that already pollute the air.

Users of inhalants are called *sniffers*. They breathe in glue, gasoline, household solvents, and aerosol sprays.

Users are starting at younger ages. The younger they are, the more harm is done to their bodies.

Users of inhalants experience it as a way to escape stress, but in actuality inhalant use increases stress. Inhalant users feel tired and not up to managing the challenges of life. They feel warm, sleepy, floating feelings like a return to mother's womb. In that euphoric mood they experience dreamy, purposeless visions. They lose coordination, alertness, and critical judgment. The most highly evolved part of the brain is blocked. They want to be held, warmed, and taken care of like babies.

In 1988 the National Institute on Drug Abuse (NIDA) released *Health Hazards of Nitrite Inhalants.*

A nitrite is a vasodilator that enlarges the passageway in blood vessels, allowing more oxygen to flow in extra blood to the brain and other tissues. As a result blood pressure can become dangerously low.

Even brief exposure to butyl or isobutyl nitrite suppresses the immune system and increases the risk of cancers and infectious diseases, including AIDS.

Amyl nitrite users are at increased risk of contracting AIDS-related Kaposi's sarcoma cancer.

Nitrites are regulated by the Food and Drug Administration. Many salt-cured meats are sources of nitrite, which bacteria break down into nitrosamine. Athletes should be careful to avoid them.

Nitrous oxide (N_2O), called laughing gas or whippets, is a psychoactive depressant drug used as an inhalant. It is used in industry in aerosol spray cans.

Nitrous oxide occurs with the breakdown of ammonium nitrate. It has been used for over a century as a light anesthetic for surgery such as in tooth extraction.

Poisoning resulting in brain damage can occur if nitrous oxide is used without enough oxygen. That can happen in a closed room while breathers are using up the oxygen supply. It can also happen to sniffers who have asthma, emphysema, lung disease, or other conditions that make it difficult to get enough oxygen.

CHAPTER 11

Coping with Stress

Your body is made up of some very complicated systems: the central nervous system involves the brain, brainstem, and spinal cord as well as the neuromuscular system that controls sports performance.

The hormonal system helps to strengthen your body and brain and to mature your performance potential. The cardiovascular system, which includes heart, lungs, and blood, is the very foundation of your aerobic capacity.

The neuromuscular system controls sports performance and can be strained by muscle tension, twitches, and tremors from drug use.

The digestive system can be stressed by having to process alcohol, cigarettes, and other drugs or too many fatty or spicy foods.

Every drug you take or chemical pollutant you inhale puts stress on all the organ systems of your body.

Sports participation can be stressful, too. Sports injuries stress your body. Winning and losing are both stressful experiences. Trying to make the team is stressful. Striving to do your personal best is stressful. Attempting to perform up to expectations can be stressful. Every sports stress that you experience puts stress on every system of your body.

Fast growth periods, with mental, emotional, and physical changes and increased needs for rest and nutriment, are stressful.

Every stress you experience causes biochemical changes in the brain and body systems. Your brain feels threatened by stress and counterattacks by sending the stress hormones, the catecholamines including adrenaline, out to fight the stress. The response is basic, even primitive, as if a lion were about to attack. Your heartbeat quickens. Blood rushes to your muscles to help you get away from the danger. Insulin is produced in larger amounts so you can metabolize extra energy.

The stress hormones are a good and ready type of unit capable of handling the normal stresses of teenage growth and maturation. Adding sports pressures, injuries, drugs and chemicals, and environmental pollution to growth stresses puts a burden on those protective forces that can eventually harm your sports abilities.

Stress can be extremely dangerous to your heart, your breathing, your processing of toxins, your energy output, your ability to handle pain, and your ability to heal injuries.

Many people respond to stress by not eating enough, which can lead to malnutrition problems and more stress. Others eat too much, becoming too heavy for their own system to manage effectively.

Stress is measurable. The body can be tested for the effects of too much stress. High triglyceride and cholesterol levels show up when people are fighting stress. Weight gain and weight loss can be caused by too much stress. Some people respond to stress by being too active, as if they could escape a threat by running from it. Some people drink alcohol or take antianxiety or other depressant drugs to slow themselves down.

Your sense of self-esteem should include taking care of your looks. Stress ages people more than anything else. It leads to wrinkling, baldness, and inability to move well or think clearly.

This chapter will suggest ways of handling stress. The previous chapters of the book have suggested ways to prevent drug stresses. You have learned of your need to cope with natural growth stresses. You have learned that 9½ hours sleep a night and eating well-balanced nutriments are especially important during adolescence and while you are taking any drug, even for medicinal purposes. Too much partying can add stress too, especially with people who pressure you to do things you know will put you at risk.

As a teenager you feel needs, desires, and pressures. Stressors are both physical and mental. You may want pleasure, understanding, solutions, glory, recognition, thrills, power, a sense of belonging to your own generation. You want a chance to try out different roles and feelings. Your actions and reactions are forming your brain.

You are exploring to find out what you can and cannot do well and what you like and do not like. You are developing skills that can be transferred to help in other situations of your life. You are getting a sense of what life-style, training schedule, and sports best fit your unique abilities and characteristics. You are learning about joy and pain and how to cope with all kinds of strong feelings. This period of your life is very intense.

This book has shown you how drugs hurt the sports community in the 1980s because athletes gave up trying to do their personal best and sought to win at all costs, risking their health and lives with drugs. Athletic events went from fair competitions to cheating competitions, using drugs to boost performance. Sports associations changed from rules based on trust to drug testing based on mistrust, because so many athletes could no longer be trusted. The role of the coach changed from training to regulating policies based on keeping athletes in line about drug use. Some pushed kids to win at all costs because their job depended on their team's success. Funding for sports was jeopardized by the end of the decade.

Some doctors went from ethical helpers to drug abusers themselves and prescription writers for profit. Many knowingly wrote unnecessary prescriptions for painkillers and antianxiety drugs that made addicts of their patients. Drug dealers too made a fast buck by selling illegal prescription drugs as well as other drugs.

The sports community was shocked with grief as many athletes died of drug overdoses and complications of use.

Student athletes went from dedication and hard work to boosting their performance with drugs, leading to lives of intense stress.

School-based programs and training camps with long hours came to be seen as the only way to get the competitive edge in sports. Many felt that drug use was the only way to cope with the intensity.

The best way to cope with the stress of sports and drugs is to take responsibility for yourself. Be careful about the choices you make. Base your decisions on as much information about risks and benefits as you can get. You need to decide how you feel about winning and losing and how you play the game.

Parents, coaches, and teammates may pressure you to work harder at sports than you can handle while you are growing. You need to decide what you yourself want. What are you doing to please other people? Trying to do something that other people want when you would rather be doing something else is a denial of who you really are. Do you know the difference? Do you play a sport because someone you care about talked you into it? How is the time spent in training affecting your grades in school?

Sports can help you accomplish some of the important tasks of your second decade of life. The development of the skills and information you need to survive in our complicated world can start with sports participation.

It is often through sports that boys and girls learn to function as members of a team. Each person learns the rules of the game so that the game goes well for everyone. You learn what you can expect and count on from others and what you have that others can rely on. Sports give you a sense of when to give and when to step aside, when to "take the ball and run with it."

Playing sports can help you be healthy and strong enough to handle the work necessary to adult living. It can help your body develop strength, flexibility, speed, endurance, and grace of movement.

Getting involved in sports can help you to make friends and keep those friendships, both by putting you in close contact with others and by learning the rules of fair play.

Physical activity can serve as an outlet for tensions and stress. You learn that doing your personal best, while meeting challenges, gives you a happy feeling of accomplishment or work satisfaction. It also gives others reason to respect you.

Everyone has good days and bad days. Doing your personal best develops a constructive attitude of acceptance of yourself when you have a down period. Growth spurts can feel down, but they do lead you up.

The rhythmic movements of sports and the excitement of competition can give you the "high" reward feelings because you have earned them. Drugs cheat the receptors. Endorphins and enkephalins help you handle the stress of physical activity and help your emotions and moods too. You can learn to have the reward feelings more often by making a wholesome life-style a habit.

Sports psychologists often recommend active rest techniques to reduce stress and improve performance. Muscular tension caused by stress keeps you from peak performance and makes you tire too soon. When you move within *active rest* your energy lasts longer and you recover faster. It takes extra energy to move tight muscles.

Active rest involves paying attention to your breathing and body rhythms to help your mind concentrate on relaxing. Sometimes a slower pace helps as you pay attention to your movements in slow motion. Your mind cannot worry when it is pleasantly involved.

Visualize yourself moving in perfect form. It can help your brain cells organize themselves toward the goal of correct movements. At the end of each day, review what you experienced during training and visualize perfect form.

Many people handle stress by keeping a journal. By writing, drawing, or even doodling in a journal they put together impressions and forces that are affecting them.

You can keep track of upsets and rewards or personal bests. Keep track of fuel expenditure: exercise; fuel storage: a balanced diet; and fuel exposure to destructive forces: drugs or pollutants.

You can log pressures and ways of relaxing that work or do not work for you. Keep a record of how much sleep you get and how you feel when you get more or less than usual.

The more you keep track of your sports experiences and issues, the more you help your brain control both your stress level and your development as an athlete.

During the night your brain will act as your private coach and think through everything you have put in your journal. Your brain will connect journal ideas with sports experiences and rearrange the connections for better performance.

You can also add pictures to your journal: photographs of yourself, your team, and successful and healthy athletes. You can then write down ways you can see yourself becoming like them.

Read descriptions of techniques that work for other athletes, and make entries in your journal about anything that inspires you. Your mental coach will inform all parts of your visualized ideal self and help you grow toward the goal. You will find yourself making the right choices, sometimes almost magically. Your brain needs your feelings and thoughts to decide whether you are being threatened or can relax.

The main task is to organize your brain. Think seriously about everything you learn and do. As you think about sports you can come up with knowledge that will help you in all areas of your life.

Remember that a well-balanced diet will give you a better chance to have what you want than any drug. You will improve your athletic performance, and even your goals.

Withdrawal symptoms and pain signals from injuries are the brain's calls for help. Withdrawal comes after many of the brain's processes have been subverted, interfered with, and modified. The help needed is a conscious and caring response. The brain is alerting the ex-user or injured athlete to take action to provide healing for all the abused nerve cells.

The ancestral wisdom of your brain assesses the losses to its body systems. It must enlist the conscious mind to help deal with the problems. Nutrients that were wasted during drug use need to be restored. Rest and reorganization of goals require focused attention. Stress needs to be reduced so that available energy resources can be directed to healing injured tissues and restoring systems to normal.

Stress can be relieved by participation in support groups that share each other's burdens. Confiding in family and friends when you are overstressed can enlist support and understanding.

Every unnatural chemical your body cells have to deal with wastes your energy and adds to your stress level. Branched chain amino acids fight stress; you need extra BCAAs for any stress you face. Drugs waste nutrients and stress your body and brain, which must work harder to compensate for the lack.

For Further Reading

Abdul-Jabbar, Kareem, and Knobler, Peter. *Giant Steps: The Autobiography of Kareem Abdul-Jabbar*. New York: Bantam, 1983.

Balch, James F. Jr. and Phyllis A. *Prescription for Nutritional Healing*. New York: Avery Publishing Group, 1990.

Cohen, Miriam. *Marijuana: Its Effects on Mind and Body*. New York: Chelsea House, 1985.

Gold, Mark S. *800-COCAINE*. New York: Bantam, 1984.

Goldman, Bob; Bush, Patricia; and Klatz, Ronald. *Death in the Locker Room: Steroids and Sports*. South Bend, IN: Icarus Press, 1984.

Hernandez, Keith, and Bryan, Mike. *If at First: A Season with the Mets*. New York: McGraw-Hill, 1986.

Klein, Gene, and Fisher, David. *First Down and a Billion: The Funny Business of Pro Football*. New York: William Morrow, 1987.

Lukas, Scott E. *Amphetamines: Danger in the Fast Lane*. New York: Chelsea House, 1985.

Margenau, Eric A. *Sports without Pressure*. New York: Gardner Press, 1990.

Micheli, Lyle J. *Sportswise: An Essential Guide for Young Athletes, Parents, and Coaches*. Boston: Houghton Mifflin, 1990.

Porter, Darrell, and Deerfield, William. *Snap Me Perfect: The Darrell Porter Story*. New York: Nelson, 1983.

Sadoff, Micky. *America Gets MADD!* Irving, TX: Mothers Against Drunk Driving, 1990.

Wachter, Oralee. *Sex, Drugs, and AIDS*. New York: Bantam Books, 1987.

Welch, Bob, with George Vecsey. *Five O'Clock Comes Too Early: A Young Man's Struggle with Alcoholism*. New York: William Morrow, 1982.

Yoder, Barbara. *The Recovery Resource Book*. New York: Simon & Schuster, 1990.

Index